Managing Pain Before It Manages You

Chapter 6

Managing Pain Before It Manages You

Third Edition

Margaret A. Caudill, MD, PhD, MPH

Foreword by Herbert Benson, MD

THE GUILFORD PRESS
New York   London

© 2009 The Guilford Press
A Division of Guilford Publications, Inc.
72 Spring Street, New York, NY 10012
www.guilford.com

Printed in the United States of America

This book is printed on acid-free paper.

Last digit is print number: 9   8   7   6   5   4   3   2

Library of Congress Cataloging-in-Publication Data

Caudill, Margaret.
    Managing pain before it manages you / Margaret A. Caudill. —
3rd ed.
        p.   cm.
    Includes bibliographical references and index.
    ISBN 978-1-59385-982-4 (pbk. : alk. paper)
    1. Pain—Popular works. I. Title.
    RB127.C384 2009
    616′.0472—dc22

                                                            2008026077

Names and identifying details of all patients' stories have been changed
to protect their anonymity. They are composites of true patient stories.

The following publishers have generously given permission to use
extended quotations from copyrighted works: The Octagon Press
(London), for excerpts from *The Pleasantries of the Incredible Mulla
Nasrudin* and *The Subtleties of the Inimitable Mulla Nasrudin and The
Exploits of the Incomparable Mulla Nasrudin* by Idries Shah (copyright
1983 by Octagon Press, Ltd.); and Beyond Words Publishing (Hillsboro,
OR), for an excerpt from *There's a Hole in My Sidewalk* by Portia
Nelson (copyright 1993 by Beyond Words Publishing).

To the patients who have instructed me in the tenacity
of the human spirit

To my family—Richard, Laura, and Paul,
Tim, Lynn, Bret, Jena, Elena, Marin, and Sabine

Contents

Foreword

Dr. Margaret Caudill has been a professional colleague for many years. She provided me with wise and successful pain management. I am deeply grateful and proud to be an associate of hers.

Dr. Caudill's expertise in pain reflects her extensive experience in wedding mind–body approaches with pain medications, therapeutic exercises, and diet. She has developed a clinically tested program recognized throughout the world. Her program for chronic pain had been scientifically proven to significantly lessen anxiety and depression, as well as anger and hostility. It diminishes the interference in life that comes with chronic pain; there is less overall distress; and in many cases the severity of pain is reduced. These improvements very frequently occur along with decreased use of pain medications, and so successful is her approach that patients on average reduce their visits to physicians by 36% for years following treatments.

Dr. Caudill has achieved these remarkable results by coupling what people can do for themselves with state-of-the-art medical treatments. The publication of *Managing Pain Before It Manages You* allows you to make use of its approach. You may also use it along with a pain regimen prescribed by your health care provider. Or you may find that your health care provider has prescribed it for you. The book is user-friendly, providing practical advice in an engaging fashion.

Those who have used this approach report that in addition to lessening their suffering from pain, they have learned how to apply its principles to other aspects of their lives. They communicate better, have a more positive attitude, and frequently achieve other elusive health goals. Overall, they report having gained more control over their lives.

Managing Pain Before It Manages You reflects the author's caring and compassion, as well as her experience and wisdom. Successful mind–body approaches require these qualities. Many patients erroneously believe that mind–body treatments mean their pain is "only in their heads." This is not what Dr. Caudill teaches. Rather, she expertly guides you through these considerations by teaching beneficial aspects of mind–body interactions to help you in improving your entire life.

I trust that your use of the approach in *Managing Pain Before It Manages You* will aid you as much as it has the many thousands who have already benefited from it.

Herbert Benson, MD
Benson–Henry Institute for Mind Body
Medicine at Massachusetts General Hospital

Acknowledgments

It is important to acknowledge the very real and crucial contributions of my colleagues Richard Schnable, Margaret Ennis, Carol Wells-Federman, and Paul Arnstein. Over the years, our dialogues and cumulative experience have created the Chronic Pain Management Program. It is impossible to distinguish where their ideas end and mine begin.

I would also like to acknowledge the invaluable support of my former colleagues at the Division of Behavioral Medicine, the Mind/Body Medical Institute, and the Arnold Pain Center at the Beth Israel Deaconess Medical Center in Boston, Massachusetts, as well as those at the Dartmouth Hitchcock Clinics and Dartmouth Hitchcock Medical Center in New Hampshire. A special thanks to Nancy L. Josephson, who is responsible for making the original material "user-friendly," as well as Barbara Watkins, Senior Editor, and Anna Brackett, Editorial Project Manager, at The Guilford Press. I wish to extend my appreciation to Eileen Stuart-Shor, the late Richard Friedman, Sharon McDonnell, Richard Slosberg, and Jay Galipeault for their support and words of encouragement over the years. Finally, a special thanks is owed to the peer advisors who have shared their experiences and support with the hundreds of patients who followed in their footsteps.

Preface

To heal does not necessarily imply to cure. It can simply
mean helping people to achieve a way of life compatible
with their individual aspirations—to restore their freedom to
make choices—even in the presence of continuing disease.
　　　　—*René Dubos*, Human Nature *(1978)*

I know I'm going to have a good day because *I know how*
to make it a good day.
　　　　　　　—Patty, after participation in this pain
　　　　　　　management program

Fourteen years after publication of this book's first edition, the treatment of
chronic pain continues to be misunderstood by the public and by many
health care professionals. While there is still no definitive cure, the past 5
years have seen an explosion in knowledge about pain, its biology, and
how best to treat it in the absence of a cure. Major developments have
occurred in three spheres. One is the study of chronic pain physiology and
of how a pain message may be kept going long after an injury. Another area
is the development of "best-practice" guidelines for diagnosis and treatment. Finally, there is the explosion of resources and information through
the Internet.

You will see these recent developments reflected in this new, third edition. Chapter 2, "Understanding Pain," updates what we know about pain
from recent research, including how pain develops and what can maintain
it. For example, complex physiological processes in the brain and spinal
cord influence the pain experience—for better or worse. This has implications for prevention and treatment. The research continues to support an
approach that engages mind, body, and social environment—all the basic
tenets of this program. This chapter also offers an overview of current
treatments for reducing chronic pain, including medications. I have attempted to distinguish drugs approved by the Food and Drug Administra-

tion (FDA) to treat pain from those used "off label" for chronic pain treatment. It is heartening to see that a number of drugs for pain other than opioids are making their way to this FDA-approved list. As I emphasize in the chapter, it's crucial to know your medications' names, dosing, and action. Create a medication list and carry it with you at all times to eliminate the potential for medication error. Finally, the discussion of treatments, in this chapter and in Appendix A, benefits from systematic reviews of research on which therapies are proven effective, which are not, and which need more study. The application of evidence-based medical findings to the area of pain medicine should bring increased consistency to treatment results and advance the cause of safe, reliable, and effective therapeutic interventions. Chapter 7, "Nutrition and Pain," has been updated to include the latest U.S. Department of Agriculture food pyramid as well as new insights into carbohydrates, oils, and supplements. Appendix A, "Common Chronic Pain Conditions," and Appendix B, "Complementary Alternative Medicine," have been updated and expanded. Appendix D is new in this edition. It contains an excellent consumer resource from the federal Agency for Healthcare Research and Quality for choosing among the nonsteroidal anti-inflammatory medications for consumers. Also new, the Internet Resources section lists some trusted Web resources for pain and health information, support groups, and research studies.

I see the possibility in the not too distant future of understanding why chronic pain occurs. With understanding will come possibilities for prevention, the effective diagnosis of pain-causing disorders, and more targeted and successful treatment. Until then, the principles of this workbook continue to be relevant for the millions who must cope with chronic pain and look within themselves for the answers—now.

Before You Begin:
How This Book Can Help You

*Thank God, I finally realized that pain may be mandatory,
but suffering is optional . . .*
—*Craig T. Nelson, actor*

We know a lot about chronic pain and are learning more every day, but many people are still left to live their lives with pain. If you have pain and have begun to see that it is not going away today (or tomorrow), then while you are waiting for the cure you might as well live life the best way you can. Practicing the skills in this book can help you get your life back.

This book has been carefully developed from years of work with brave people experiencing pain. If you have begun reading this book, you have probably been living with pain for some time. You may have a painful disease for which there is no cure, or you may have experienced the tremendous frustration of trying to explain to doctors that your pain is real and it is persisting, even though they can't find a cause for it. They may have told you that all your tests have come back negative, that there is no medical explanation for your continued suffering, that surgery should have worked, or something similar. They may have also suggested, directly or indirectly, that your condition is the result of emotional stress—or perhaps even that "it's all in your head"—and that you should consider seeing a psychologist.

As if this weren't bad enough, you must return home and face your anxious loved ones, who have been hoping against hope for a "miracle cure" so that you and they can resume something like normal family life. You must now tell them that your condition is unchanged and that you have exhausted all medical help. If you have not returned to work but run into colleagues, you must explain to them that you have not been on vacation and politely tolerate their unsupportive comments ("Aren't you better *yet*?") or their suggestions for home remedies (snake livers, copper bracelets, etc.). In short, you may feel abandoned, panicky, and utterly alone.

This book is for you if you can say, "I have chronic pain, it's real, and I need help." But you don't have to be at the end of your rope to use this book. The skills it describes can also help you get more out of your ongoing medical treatment. For you at this time, pain may be mandatory, but suffering is optional. And you are definitely not alone.

This book is also for you if you are the relative or friend of a person in chronic pain. It may increase your own understanding of the pain experience, or it could be an important gift to that special person. Finally, this book is for you if you are a health care professional; it can be a valuable resource for you and your patients who must live in pain.

Is the following story familiar to you?

A Common Story

Pat entered the new specialist's office, tired and apprehensive at the prospect of describing her pain once again to a stranger. No one ever seemed to listen when she tried to explain what it was like to wake up and go to bed day after day in pain. Every day it became more of an effort to take care of herself and her family. Her children wondered, "Gee, Mom, what's wrong with you? Why won't they fix it?" Two nights ago her husband—frustrated, she knew, at his own sense of powerlessness—had snapped, "Why can't you just ignore it?" She remembered her family physician's words at her last visit: "There is nothing else I can do. You have chronic pain and must learn to live with it." She had cried all the way home. Her doctor, however, had also given her the name of a pain specialist who worked with people in chronic pain and had been successful in helping them. She didn't like this alternative at all. But after spending thousands of dollars, experiencing medication side effects, undergoing unsuccessful surgery, and seeing six consultants, she was no closer to getting rid of the pain.

So now here she was waiting for someone else to give her bad news. The pain management doctor, however, asked types of questions she had not heard before—questions about her experience of pain: Had she ever noticed that her pain increased with certain activities, particularly when she ignored the early spasms warning her to stop? Did she find that if she was anxious or upset about family or financial matters, her pain flared up as well? Was she more short-tempered than she used to be? Did she cry more easily? Was she experiencing non-pain symptoms—like shortness of breath, palpitations, fatigue, or sleep problems? Pat answered yes to all of these questions.

The pain specialist told Pat that her pain was real—it was absolutely not "all in her head"—but that medical science did not yet know how to take it away. She was one of millions of people caught in a tangled web of chronic pain. However, many of Pat's symptoms were manageable, because they were the results of ignoring the limits placed on her by the pain. By identifying new ways of working with and relating to her pain, she could feel less helpless, less hopeless, and more in control. She could even feel more productive and better about herself

---

just by practicing certain techniques and modifying her daily routine in a way that allowed her to take her discomfort into consideration. The threads of Pat's pain web could in fact be untangled and rewoven into a safety net if she followed this program.

Pat was still a little skeptical, but she decided to give it a try. She felt that at this point she had nothing to lose and everything to gain.

This book describes the program that helped Pat. It can help you too.

How Effective Is the Program?

Like Pat, are you still a little skeptical?

The program presented in this book has been proven effective in helping people in chronic pain improve their quality of life. My colleagues and I first reported this in a paper published in the scientific journal *The Clinical Journal of Pain* (7: 305–310, 1991). Before our patients participated in a pain management program identical to the one in this book, they averaged 12 doctor visits a year. After participating, the patients did not need to see their doctors as frequently (down to seven visits per year), and doctor visits remained decreased for up to 2 years after the end of the program. Furthermore, the patients reported less depression, less anxiety, lower pain severity, and less interference of pain in their activities. They also noted increases in their feelings of being in control and in their general activity levels.

My colleagues and I believe that this program works because it helps people increase their ability to manage, function, and cope with pain. Belief in your ability to manage, function, and cope with challenges is called "self-efficacy." Our research published in the journal *Pain* (81: 483–491, 1999) shows that your sense of self-efficacy influences how much your pain depresses or disables you. Practicing the skills in this book will help you gain control over the pain.

What Can You Expect?

The program described here does not offer any "miracle cures." It also does not promise to make your life exactly the way it was before you had the pain. However, no one is suggesting that you should just passively endure your pain. If you learn and use the skills in this book, you can expect to become active and involved in your life again. You can do this in a way that will minimize pain increases and reduce the distress of having a pain problem. By becoming involved in your pain treatment, you become part of the solution to the problem.

What's Involved?

This pain management program will help you understand what chronic pain is and why certain treatments may have been prescribed for you in the past. You will be asked to explore your pain experience by tracking it on a daily basis. You can use a diary form included in this book to record how what you do now affects your pain. Later, you can record the effects on your pain of doing things differently. This is a way of beginning to untangle the pain web you have been caught in. You will be given many opportunities to reflect on how you wish to live each day. Many old habits that served you well in the past may not work now that you are challenged by pain.

Many ways to reduce stress will be presented. These will include breath exercises, techniques that bring about a particular physical reaction called the "relaxation response," stretching techniques, and body awareness exercises. In addition, this book will show you how to become more active with less pain by learning how to pace and plan your daily activities. The book will help you explore methods of moving when you are in pain and how to use breathing to reduce the tension of pain during movement. Ways of using nutrition to your advantage will also be discussed.

Moreover, this book can teach you skills for coping with the sadness, anxiety, or anger you may be experiencing. This includes methods for communicating your needs clearly and expressing yourself effectively to those around you, including your health care provider. Finally, you can learn techniques for problem solving and for beginning to plan a new life in spite of the pain. You will then be ready to reweave the untangled threads of your old pain web into a safety net.

This program is meant to empower you to act in your own best interests. In fact, by deciding to read this far, you have been learning to exercise choice. You may at any time put down this book and stop the process, but choosing to go on can open many doors for you. Will you stay where you are, feeling trapped and misunderstood, or will you begin to evaluate and understand how your pain can be modified? Will you continue to feel that you are at the mercy of your pain, or will you begin to live with hope? You do have choices.

How to Use This Book

This program has been used by many people who feel just like you do. They have, like you, bravely made the first step toward managing their pain by picking up this book. Whether you are reading it by yourself or with a group of other people in pain, you can be assured that your struggles are universal ones. Reading the patients' stories presented throughout the book may also help you to feel less lonely in your work.

Most people find that they make the best use of the book by reading about a chapter a week, but everyone should set his or her own pace. Allow enough time to answer all the questions in each chapter and complete all the exploration tasks (see the next section). More skills and techniques will be added as you read through the book. Many of the tasks do not require you to make extra time in your schedule for them; they simply require you to pay attention to how you do the things you already do. Some of the skills and techniques, such as the ones in the chapters on attitudes and communication, may take a little more time.

Keep in mind that there is no need for you to finish all 10 chapters in 10 weeks. Research studies with self-changers and smokers suggest that it takes at least 10 weeks to begin to change behavior and that 6 months of sustained action are required to progress to maintenance of these changes. Research also shows that real change and therefore real benefits take place only when people act upon the written word. If you are really in doubt about the benefits of working with this book, just reading it may be what you need to do at this time. If you are ready to change the way you feel and to improve your life in pain then it's essential to actually carry out the exercises in this book.

Special Features of This Book

This book offers a number of special features to help you. These include chapter summaries, exploration tasks, supplementary reading lists, free audio downloads of guided relaxations, appendices, and end-of-book worksheets and other materials.

At the end of each chapter, you will find a *summary* of its key points. You may find it helpful to read the summary first —a preview of coming attractions, so to speak. Reviewing the summary after reading the chapter is useful for picking up certain points or aspects that you may have forgotten.

Most chapters include *exploration tasks*. Complete each set of tasks before you move on to the next chapter. These tasks are designed to reinforce what you've learned in the chapter. They ask you to apply the chapter's skills to your particular situation and put them into practice. This is where the real learning is done. If you are working on a chapter a week, the exploration tasks will clarify what skills you should be practicing at any particular time.

There are *supplementary reading lists* at the end of most chapters. You can use these reading materials to help you develop your coping skills further. The combined contents of these lists (and a few additional resources) are presented in the Bibliography.

To help you learn and practice the relaxation response techniques in Chapter 3, you can download *audio of guided relaxations* that I have recorded. These are free and available from the publisher's website (*www.guilford.com/managepain*). Have this book handy when you go to download; you will be asked to type in a password from the book. Just follow the directions on the website.

You can find other helpful resources in the *appendices*. Appendix A, "Common Chronic Pain Conditions," is a review of observations I have made on various chronic pain syndromes. It can serve as a resource for support groups or for further treatment recommendations in some instances. Appendix B, "Complementary Alternative Medicine," discusses other therapies used for pain treatment. Appendix C, "Working Comfortably," was written by a former patient to help those who must work at a computer terminal. It has important recommendations to prevent injuries or relapses. The Internet Resources section is an index of Internet addresses for a variety of reliable sources for health and pain information. Appendix D is the consumer guide to *Choosing Pain Medicine for Osteoarthritis* from the U.S. Agency for Healthcare Research and Quality.

In Appendix E and at the end of the book are *worksheets* and other materials that can be photocopied by purchasers of this book for personal use only (see copyright page for details). To facilitate photocopying, the second set has been perforated and can be easily removed. The worksheets include a pain diary sheet (see Chapter 1 for an explanation of its use); a medication list (see Chapter 2); a relaxation response diary sheet (see Chapter 3); an increasing activities worksheet (see Chapter 4); a worksheet for monitoring your self-talk, emotions, and other responses to stressful events (see Chapter 5); a food diary sheet (see Chapter 7); and a weekly feedback sheet for giving your health care professional information about your pain experience (see Chapter 8).

Additional materials include (1) a "Do Not Disturb" sign that can be copied and hung on your door to prevent interruptions during your practice of relaxation response techniques and (2) a letter to your health care professional, which I encourage you to copy and take to your next visit. It explains how your health care provider can help you use the information in this book, and it can help enlist his or her participation in this program if you have picked up the book on your own.

A Final Note

The solutions offered in this book are for real people living in the real world. The skills and techniques are practical, and the recommendations are based on years of working with people in pain just like you. You are encouraged to read and reread carefully even statements that you may find disagreeable or distressing. The last thing you may want to hear is that it is possible to live in pain or that after reading this book you will not necessarily be pain free. I do understand that it is not your choice to be in pain and that your life has been changed by your pain. These recommendations for working with your pain and rebuilding your life are not made lightly. They are made because I have seen that, with help, people are able to live with and even rise above their pain in remarkable ways. You can be productive, can enjoy life's pleasures, and can even fulfill some dreams if you apply what you read in this book to your pain problem. I hope that this will be a positive new beginning for you. Welcome to the program!

1

Beginning to Take Control
of Your Pain

You may still have doubts about whether you can ever enjoy life again while you are in chronic pain. Nevertheless, let's at least explore how living a life of quality with chronic pain is possible. The keys are to take ownership of your pain (and this doesn't mean blaming yourself for it), determine exactly what your problems are as a result of the pain, and reassess your goals in the light of this information. This chapter gives you your first set of tools for beginning to take control of your pain: diary keeping and goal setting. To begin, look at the first of the three keys: accepting ownership of your pain.

Accepting Ownership of Your Pain

Your problem is that you are in pain and the pain won't go away. Defining the problem in this way is an important first step; before you can do anything about your pain, you need to acknowledge that it exists.

You may also feel inclined at this point to blame others for your pain. You may feel that your doctors have failed you by not finding and curing the source of the pain or at least by not making you feel better. You may believe that your loved ones are not doing anything to help you or are showing a lack of understanding or empathy about your problem. You may even feel that society is to blame for causing the situation that put you in pain in the first place or for not making it easier for you to seek help.

The fact that you may be sad, angry, or anxious about the disruption of your whole life as a result of the pain experience is both understandable and normal. Under these circumstances, it may be very tempting to feel that others are to blame for the pain and ought to be responsible for taking it away. Indeed, many people in pain put their whole lives on hold waiting for others—their physicians, their families, or society—to do just this. The difficulty with this is that wanting to give away both the pain and the responsibility for coping with it only prolongs your feelings of powerlessness. If your pain is not going away anytime soon—and this is the very nature of chronic pain—then taking on responsibility for living with it begins to return control of your life to you. If you can adopt an attitude of "ownership" of the pain problem, you have the potential for gaining the upper hand over it. Although you may need assistance from your health care professional, your family, and society, it is ultimately your task and yours alone to untangle yourself from your pain web.

You may now be thinking: "Oh, great. So I'm responsible for my pain, huh? I'm to blame? That's what everybody's been saying—or at least hinting—all along. I feel bad and guilty enough as it is." That is not what is meant here at all. As you probably already know, self-blame and guilt can be paralyzing emotions. They can make you feel so bad and worthless there's no point in doing anything at all. Accepting ownership of your pain, on the other hand, means acknowledging that you *are* a worthwhile person, that there *is* a point in doing something, and that you *do* have choices. It is very different from blaming yourself.

Chronic pain is complex, with many origins and treatments. It is grossly misunderstood. This book will provide you with the information you need to move forward. Even though your life will be different from the way it was before the pain, you can change some aspects of the pain. You can learn to work with other aspects so that they cause you less distress. Your task will be difficult—but not impossible.

Determining Exactly What Your Problems Are

Order and simplification are the first steps toward mastery of a subject—the actual enemy is the unknown.
—*Thomas Mann*, The Magic Mountain *(1924)*

The Importance of Tracking Your Pain Levels

One important way to gain control over your pain is to record it. This allows you to see what (for instance, activities, weather, tension, and sleeplessness) increases or decreases your pain. Recording should be done three times a day, at regular times that are convenient for you. For example, you might write down your pain level when you wake up, after lunch, and then again at bedtime. Such consistency is important, because if you record your pain only when you are aware of it, you won't necessarily notice when your pain level changes. Recording the pain at regular intervals will allow you to discover that there are patterns in your pain experience over time. Becoming aware of these patterns will help you to determine what makes the pain better or worse, what helps and what hurts.

Many people are resistant at first to the idea of tracking their pain, and you may be one of them. Not only are you in pain to begin with, but it's an additional hassle to have to record all this stuff—and three times a day! "Why do I have to do this? It's not fair!" you may say. Perhaps the following story will help.

Paula was very angry at the thought of keeping track of her pain levels. Her back hurt and she already knew she was in pain. Why did she have to write it down three times a day, every day?

At first, Paula was so miserable that recording the pain just made her realize how bad she felt. Gradually, she realized how much she denied the pain in her back and how it prevented her from doing anything productive or pleasurable. Not only had she given up working outside the home, but she barely kept up with the household chores. Her house certainly wasn't as clean as it used to be. Even worse, she was irritable toward her husband and yelled at her children. She rarely saw her friends and really didn't care anymore about going out. Somehow this just wasn't the way Paula wanted to live.

Then Paula began to see how she pushed herself throughout the day and collapsed at night. Her back was stiff when she awoke, and the pain gradually increased during the day. What was causing the increase? Was it the fact that she "pushed, crashed, and burned" on a regular basis? Would pacing her activities help? Did this contribute to her feeling out of control? Slowly the answers became clear.

Over time, Paula saw that keeping track of her pain levels helped her learn more about the connection between her pain and her activities, what she did and how she did it. She was able to incorporate the skills she was learning for pain management into her daily routine and was eventually able to decrease the pain, bringing it more under her control.

If you don't think that recording your pain will be a chore, that's great. If you do, consider this: You have done your best in your current situation, and it still hasn't been effective in controlling your pain. Recording your pain levels can help you determine where you might be stuck and point you in the right direction. You can't count on remembering exactly what your pain feels like under all conditions over a long period of time. So give the recording method a shot—it just might work for you. Remember: *What you know, you can master.*

Keeping a Pain Diary

An effective way of tracking your pain is to keep the pain diary worksheet provided at the end of this book. There is a sample of a completed pain diary form, along with a blank pain diary form that can be copied.

In your pain diary it is important to keep track of both the physical (bodily) sensations of pain and any unpleasant emotions associated with the pain—the emotional response. "Physical sensation" refers to the aching, stabbing, burning, pounding, tightness, and other bodily sensations you may feel. In the pain diary, "Emotional response" refers to the unpleasant or negative emotions associated with your pain and is a measure of suffering—for example, frustration, anxiety, anger, or sadness. Such unpleasant emotions are often associated with thinking such thoughts as "This [pain] will never go away," "It's not fair!," "I'm useless," and "My life is worthless." This can make you and your pain feel even worse.

Note that the word "feel" can be used to describe both physical/body sensations and emotional/mind reactions. This dual meaning can be confusing when you try to describe the pain experience to yourself and to the outside world. I began asking patients in pain to make the distinction between the two meanings years ago, at the last session of my very first pain group. The patients were talking about how great they felt and yet their "pain level" was only slightly lower than what they had recorded 10 weeks earlier. I was puzzled and I asked them to help me understand what had happened. They explained, "Oh we still have pain [the physical sensation], but we feel so much better [the emotional response] about it. We aren't helpless now and we know what to do when our pain increases. We're in control, not the pain!"

Most health care workers do not make this distinction and do not understand the dual meaning that pain can have. They make the mistake of using one scale, a single rating of pain when they ask patients "What pain level are you experiencing?" If you get asked this question, be sure to clarify what you mean. It will assist you in getting the appropriate medicine at the correct dose for your specific symptom.

The fact is that a lot more can be done about the emotional response to chronic pain than about the physical experience. And this can make you feel a whole lot better about dealing with chronic pain, as it did with our patients. You can begin by getting in touch with how you experience your pain, both physically and emotionally. You may find that at any one time you have more emotional than physical feelings related to your pain or just the opposite, more physical than emotional feelings. It will take some time and practice to see the difference, but it will be worth the effort. Some of the exercises in the next few chapters will help you to separate these feelings.

I recommend that you continue to fill out the pain diary form for at least 3 months. You can stop once your pain levels appear stable and you are feeling better and in more control of your response to the pain. You can always start again if your pain worsens, a new symptom occurs, or you are tracking your response to a new treatment. Here are more detailed instructions for keeping your pain diary.

Instructions

1. Record your pain level on the pain diary form (see pp. 216–217) three times a day at regular intervals—for example, morning, noon, and bedtime.

2. Begin each recording by writing the date and time.

3. In the space under "Describe situation," note what activity(-ies) you were engaged in during the previous 4–6 hours. For example, were you watching TV, shopping, sitting at a computer, or cleaning the house or garage all day?

4. Rate the intensity of your physical sensation (and its effect on your activities) by using the numbers in the chart below. Write a one-word description of your physical sensation. Separately, rate your emotional response using the numbers below. Write a one-word description of your emotional response.

The numbers you give to your physical sensation and emotional response do not have to increase or decrease together. For example, you can have a high level of pain sensation and yet not necessarily suffer emotionally because of it. This will become more apparent as you proceed through the book and learn new pain management skills. Give ratings on a scale from 0 to 10 as follows:

Ratings	Physical sensation/activities	Emotional/negative feelings response
0	No painful physical sensation No alteration in activities	No negative emotional response
1–4	Low intensity of physical sensation, minimal effect on activities	Minimal/low level of negative emotions (frustrated, disappointed)
5–6	Moderate intensity of physical sensation associated with increased body tension; moderate restriction of activities	Moderate intensity of negative emotions (anxious, sad, irritable)
7–8	Significant pain sensation associated with difficulty moving; decreased activities	Significant negative emotions, making it hard to engage in activities (fearful, angry, depressed)
9–10	Severe pain sensation associated with inability to move; able to participate in only minimal activities; bedridden	Severe depression, anxiety, or despair associated with significant impairment of thinking

It may take several weeks to establish what the numbers mean for you. This is quite normal. Pain is a personal experience, and you'll only be rating your own experience. (If you have particular or continuing difficulty, however, see the "Rating Your Pain" exercise under "Listening to Your Body" in Chapter 4.)

5. Record any medication or action you take to help alleviate the pain. For example, if you soak in a hot tub, go for a walk, stretch, or take two aspirin, record the fact.

6. At the end of each day, add the numbers from the three ratings for physical sensation together and average them by dividing the total by three. You will then have one daily physical sensation rating. Do the same for your ratings of emotional response. Making a graph of the numbers for different times of day and for the daily averages can help you see the pain patterns more clearly over the weeks and months during which you develop your program of self-management.

The pain diary is intended for your benefit and self-exploration. You can change it if that would be helpful. For example, you can record pain in two separate areas of the body or you can record your emotional responses to life as well as your emotional responses to pain. The pain diary can also be an important source of information when you see your health care professional, particularly when the two of you are tracking symptom flare-ups or your response to treatment.

Noting Variations in Your Pain

If you find yourself rating your physical sensation with the same number three times a day, 7 days a week, examine your pain more closely. It is common for people in pain to think of their pain as overwhelming, unvarying, and unremitting. However, both physical sensation and emotional response vary; they rarely remain constant for days and weeks at a time. This natural variation is the result of your attention shifting from one thing to another. Mood, fatigue, muscle tension, and other factors also influence the pain experience from moment to moment. The brain is the final judge of sensory input and the center of emotional response. It tends to pay the most attention to changing levels of sensation or events. It quickly becomes bored with constant sounds, pain, and so forth, whether from outside or inside the body. As a result the pain and the awareness of pain will vary as well.

For example, if you go into a room with a fan running overhead you may be aware of the sound when you first enter; after a short period of time, however, you will "forget" the sound. If the fan shuts off, you may pay attention again, noticing the absence of the sound for a few seconds. Likewise, you may not be aware of the pressure of your back against a chair as you sit reading this, but now that I've pointed it out, you are suddenly aware of it. This awareness, too, will suddenly disappear after a few seconds as you read on.

You can make use of the brain's short attention span for constant sensation; it is a way of altering the pain experience. Such techniques will be discussed in later chapters.

What's Next?

You are most likely going to feel worse for the next few weeks. You may say, "Oh, no! I thought this program was supposed to make me feel better, not worse." Well, don't panic just yet. This program begins by helping you identify what you have been experiencing, both physically and emotionally. If you begin to feel worse, it is not necessarily because the disease causing the pain is getting worse; it is more likely because you are bringing your pain experience into consciousness. Bringing the pain to the front row of your attention can alter your sensitivity to it. Remember this for future reference: Changing your awareness changes the pain experience.

Many people use denial to cope with their pain. This may work for short-term problems. Long-term problems usually require conscious solutions. Awareness of your pain allows you to engage in activities in a way that will not make your pain worse. You will be asked to increase your awareness of your daily thoughts, experiences, and interactions throughout this program. You will learn how to distract yourself from the pain; however, this will be a conscious action, completely under your control, and free from any harmful side effects. It is a process that occurs in multiple steps and takes time. You are now just beginning the first step.

Setting Goals

People in pain often feel scattered, adrift, unfocused, and unsuccessful. Because pain restricts activities, it can become difficult to accomplish anything. No doubt, you find yourself unable to do all that you had hoped. When meaningful activity is taken away because of chronic pain, you suffer even more. Keeping a pain diary is one way to start focusing your life; it brings order to this "big unknown" (the pain) and helps you know how best to cope with it.

Another way is to set goals—a first step in slowly bringing order, success, and accomplishment back to your life. Setting goals will also help you commit to this program. But if you are not used to setting goals, it can be tricky. The key is to set *achievable* goals—that is, goals you can accomplish. This is particularly important when you are learning how to live with your pain. You don't need to feel like a failure any more than you perhaps already do. There are ways to set goals so that you cannot fail. When you take the goal-setting process slowly and easily, each small success helps you reach higher.

Let's start by choosing three goals you would like to achieve through working with this book. The goals should be short-term ones that can be accomplished in 2 to 3 months. Use the following criteria to develop your goals:

Goal-Setting Criteria

1. *A goal should be measurable.* How will you know when the goal has been reached?

2. *A goal should be realistic.* Is it possible to achieve, even in pain?

3. *A goal should be behavioral.* Does it involve specific actions or steps to take?

4. *A goal should be "I"-centered.* Are *you* the one engaging in the actions or behaviors to be measured?

5. *A goal should be desirable.* Do you want the results enough to put forth the effort?

Cindy's goal was to feel less stressed in 4 weeks. It sounded reasonable, but what exactly did it mean? Was the goal "feeling less stressed" measurable? What was "feeling stressed"? What did she mean by "less stressed"? What changes in behavior were needed to accomplish the goal? In other words, what specific actions or steps did Cindy need to take? Her success would be left to chance if she didn't answer these questions. And leaving it to chance would not guarantee her success; it might even make it unlikely.

Cindy reworked her goal and decided that to her, "feeling stressed" meant feeling muscle tightness in the back of her neck. She wanted to be able to lessen this tension. If she could do that, maybe her headaches would be helped too. Now she could make a list of what she could do (*behaviors*) to accomplish her *measurable* and *desirable* goal—reduce tension in the neck and reduce the number of headaches.

Cindy decided that she would swim three times a week, take a stretch break from her work at the computer every hour for 60 seconds (see Chapter 4), and practice a relaxation response technique (see Chapter 3) once a day. She thus made her goal *"I"-centered* (she, not someone else, would be taking these steps), *behavioral* (there were specific, clear action steps to take), and *realistic* (these steps would be relatively easy for her to take).

After Cindy had worked toward her goal for a while, she could see for herself whether the tension was decreased in her neck and whether this was influencing her headaches. Her success was not left to chance but was the result of a conscious effort on her part.

Goal-Setting Exercise

Now list three pain management goals that you would like to accomplish in the next 2 to 3 months. Make them achievable in each of the five ways described above. If you don't yet know what steps to take to accomplish the goals, leave those blank for now; come back to them after reading more of this book.

Let's use Cindy's goal as an example:

1. **Goal:** <u>Decrease tension in the back of the neck and decrease headaches.</u>

   Steps to take to reach that goal:

   A. <u>Swim three times a week.</u>

   B. <u>Take frequent stretch breaks at the computer.</u>

   C. <u>Practice a relaxation response technique once a day.</u>

Now it's your turn.

1. Goal: _____

Steps to take to reach that goal:

A. _____

B. _____

C. _____

2. Goal: _____

Steps to take to reach that goal:

A. _____

B. _____

C. _____

3. Goal: _____

Steps to take to reach that goal:

A. _____

B. _____

C. _____

Setting goals now is a way of making a commitment to this self-management program. If you find yourself confused or resistant, ask yourself why. Have you been clear enough in defining what you want? Do you want something that you can't achieve at this time? Is there a part—even a small part—of what you want that is achievable? Don't be surprised if you find yourself feeling sad, angry, or frustrated with this exercise, particularly if there are things you wish to do but can't. The ability to be flexible and identify other goals that are available to you, in spite of the pain, can be very rewarding. Once again, you do have choices. Setting goals is a step toward identifying those options.

Congratulate yourself for having the courage and determination to begin this process. You have begun to gain control over your life!

Summary

- Taking ownership of your pain is the first step in gaining control over it.
- Recording your pain in the pain diary helps you track your physical pain sensation and your emotional response.
- Tracking your pain helps you see what increases or decreases it. This can tell you exactly what your problems are and help you solve them.

- Acknowledging your pain may make you feel worse—temporarily. However, you can learn to distract yourself consciously from pain.
- Setting achievable goals is important in bringing accomplishment back into your life.
- Achievable goals are measurable, realistic, behavioral, "I"-centered, and desirable.

Exploration Tasks

1. When your pain gets worse, list the things that you do now to make it better:

_____

_____

_____

_____

2. Draw a picture of you and your pain. Use crayons or colored pencils. No black-and-white pictures, please! This artwork need not be displayed unless you want it to be, but it can be an important exercise to look at pain in a nonverbal way.

Use this space to draw yourself and your pain:

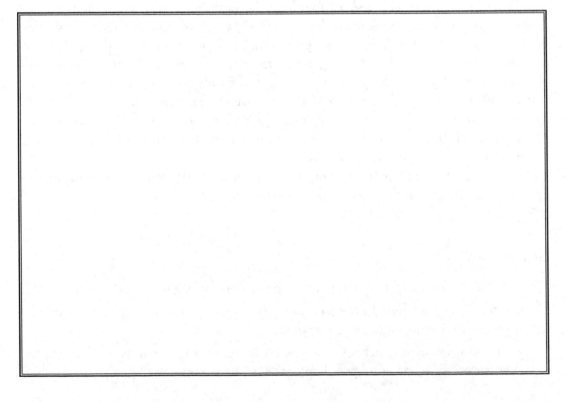

2

Understanding Pain

Pain, like fever, is a symptom. It is also an important and necessary component of the human experience. Let's take a look at the various meanings of pain:

- *Biologically,* pain is a signal that the body has been harmed.
- *Psychologically,* pain is experienced as emotional suffering.
- *Behaviorally,* pain alters the way a person moves and acts.
- *Cognitively,* pain calls for thinking about its meaning, its cause, and possible remedies.
- *Spiritually,* pain has been a reminder of mortality.
- *Culturally,* pain has been used to test people's fortitude or to force their submission.

Pain is a complex process, and the pain signal can be magnified, minimized, and reinterpreted by a person's experiences, both past and present.

Pain can be divided into two major categories—acute and chronic—based on how long it lasts and the underlying cause.

Acute Pain

Acute pain is time limited and lasts long enough for healing to begin, generally from 24 hours to 10 days. It warns us of tissue injury or harm. Acute pain is associated with physical trauma such as abnormal crushing, stretching, or tearing of tissue. Acute pain can also come from tissue irritation or inflammation in response to infection, injury, or disease.

Inflammation is the body's way to fight infection or heal tissue after injury. The normal inflammation process involves cells in the body that release chemicals that signal the nerves, muscles, and blood vessels to begin the healing process.

When you are injured, cells in the damaged area release chemicals that irritate the pain nerves. Pain nerves send their signal to the spinal cord, and you perceive pain. This makes you aware of the injury. Other chemicals released by damaged cells cue other responses to injury. Muscle spasms are triggered, and these protect the area from movement. Blood vessels in the surrounding tissue constrict, reducing bleeding. White blood cells and connective tissue cells start cleaning up and repairing the damage.

There are also special pain nerves deep inside the body that detect stretch or blockage of blood flow to vital organs. These sensory nerves alert us to blockage of the bowels or the blood vessels of the heart or bleeding into the head. These special pain nerves connect to the spinal cord close to where peripheral pain nerves also connect. As a result internal pain may be felt first in the arms or legs. For example, arm pain is associated with a heart attack, shoulder pain is associated with a gallbladder attack, and thigh pain is associated with bladder irritation.

Here are some conditions associated with acute pain:

- *A burn*. We touch the hot iron, and instantly the hand is withdrawn. The hot iron has stimulated pain receptors in the hand. It is too much heat for the tissue to be exposed to safely. A reflex to move the hand out of harm's way occurs automatically, and then we rush to the sink to run cool water over the burned area.

- *Appendicitis*. The pain from an infected appendix is a more complicated process because it involves inflammation in an internal organ, the appendix. At first the person with appendicitis may be aware only of a vague stomachache in the area around the belly button. Appetite may decrease or fever may be present. As the appendix becomes more inflamed, the pain is localized to the right lower quadrant of the abdomen, and the muscles above the appendix spasm. The pain serves as a warning that something is wrong and drives a person to search for relief, usually through surgical removal of the appendix.

- *Labor pains*. The pain during childbirth is caused by stretching of the cervix around the baby's head and contractions of the uterine muscle. Although the pain receptors in the cervix respond to the abnormal stretching, the woman's experience of labor pain can be modified by distraction, massage, and supportive coaching and by blocking the pain pathways with anesthetics.

- *Cancer pain (acute)*. The pain associated with cancer is usually the result of the cancer invading tissues and blocking normal organ functions or pressing directly on nerves.

In all of these examples, pain is a warning symptom that triggers a person to act. These actions can be automatic, such as pulling the hand away from a hot iron, or purposeful, such as seeking help. Anxiety and fear are normal emotional responses to pain that further motivate a person to seek relief. But the situation in which pain occurs may modify these emotional responses. Modified emotions, in turn, can modify the experience of the pain, as seen in the pain of childbirth.

Acute pain is an important symptom to heed. But once treatment begins there is no advantage to withholding pain relief. Unrelieved pain after surgery can cause complications (pneumonia and immobility), and in patients with cancer it can cause unnecessary suffering. Supporting these observations is a major education initiative in the United States to advocate for timely and adequate treatment of acute pain and cancer pain.

Chronic Pain

Chronic pain lasts longer than acute pain and is caused by a different set of conditions.

At least three conditions are associated with chronic pain and help explain its long duration. First, there is a painful, underlying chronic disease; second, the pain nerves are damaged; and third, there are changes in the brain or spinal cord that control the pain message, increasing its volume and duration.

Some chronic pain problems result from diseases that cause chronic inflammation or irritation. In diseases such as rheumatoid arthritis, lupus arthritis, and osteoarthritis there is an ongoing release of irritating substances. These substances trigger acute pain mechanisms but do so in a way that lasts for months and years. This type of pain may be relieved almost completely if the underlying disease responds to treatment or even by joint replacement when the joint can no longer function well.

Another cause of chronic pain has only become better understood in the past two decades. In this case, chronic pain arises from damage to the pain system itself. Like a broken fire alarm that continues to clang when there is no fire, pain may persist long after an injury has healed. Some diseases, injuries, and cancer drug or radiation therapies can cause nerve damage. And in some circumstances we now believe there may be a genetic tendency for the pain response to go awry. The symptom of pain, originally a warning, now becomes the problem. It doesn't go away.

In these circumstances the pain's source or cause may be difficult to explain at first. There are often delays in making the diagnosis that can result in multiple biological, psychological, and social consequences. Here are some problems associated with pain system damage:

- Nerve pain associated with diabetes (diabetic neuropathy)
- Pain after shingles (postherpetic neuralgia)
- Fibromyalgia
- Chronic pelvic pain
- Chronic bladder pain (interstitial cystitis)
- Postsurgical back pain

Chronic pain may last indefinitely. It may never completely go away, or it may be intermittent. With chronic intermittent pain, people may have pain-free periods of weeks or months alternating with extended periods of daily pain. Examples include migraine headaches, cluster headaches, muscle tension headaches, and irritable bowel syndrome.

The Experience of Chronic Pain

With chronic pain, the pain experience may be magnified because of its long duration with no relief. This experience may be modified by the environment (changes in weather), expectations ("If I have pain, I must be doing something wrong"), a search for meaning ("Why me?"), and/or cultural beliefs ("No pain, no gain"). Your perceptions (beliefs, attitudes, moods) greatly affect your experience of chronic pain.

Although there may be no clear explanation for your chronic pain, you are understandably driven biologically and psychologically to resolve the problem. Remember that the presence of pain and the pressure to act on its presence are established in a very old and primitive part of the brain. When the pain system is doing its job, it is a warning of danger and harm. When the system is overloaded or damaged it can be a source of physical and emotional stress. As a result, you may suffer even more symptoms (such as fatigue, muscle tension, and insomnia). These additional symptoms are the result of the stress you suffer from chronic pain.

For months or years, you have been experiencing the constant stimulus of pain. Biologically, you have had to live with a signal that usually requires the utmost urgency and attention. Psychologically, you may feel anxious, depressed, and abandoned. Behaviorally, you may have become less sociable; you may have withdrawn from activities or the company of others. Cognitively, you may think yourself inadequate to meet this challenge, or you may be at your wits' end not knowing what to do. Spiritually, you may feel beaten down and abandoned. And culturally, you may be fighting beliefs or expectations about how you should suffer.

It's important for you to understand what chronic pain is, what it isn't, and what we think keeps it going. Your enemy is the unknown. Understanding the pain process can bring you closer to its mastery. You can begin to do that by keeping a pain diary, which helps you establish what the pain experience is like for you.

Now that you've had a chance to learn a little about acute and chronic pain, take a minute to read the following. This is a story common to many who end up with chronic pain. See whether you can identify both the acute and chronic phases of the process.

Sarah was a very active 31-year-old English professor who liked to garden, dance, and ride horses in her spare time. One day as she bent to turn her compost pile, she experienced searing pain down her right leg, causing her to limp as she walked away. She took it easy for a week, stopped exercising, and didn't ride her horse to see whether the pain would get better. It didn't. She then went to her doctor. An examination showed that Sarah had lost the reflexes in her right leg. A computerized axial tomography (CAT) scan revealed a herniated disc in her lower back. She was referred to a neurosurgeon, who recommended surgery.

By now Sarah's pain was constantly sending knife-like sensations into her leg and down the calf to her foot. It was impossible for her to find a comfortable position in which to sleep, and the constant pain was always on her mind. She had nightmares of having surgery and being confined to a wheelchair for the rest of her life. She was anxious and frightened. She took a medical leave of absence from her job because the pain would not allow her to carry out her teaching responsibilities.

Sarah spent 3 anxious and painful weeks hoping that the pain would subside; when it didn't, she made the decision to have the surgery. It went well, and even though Sarah was sore and tight from the incision, her leg was already feeling better than it had in weeks. The pain from her incision was made tolerable by pain medication. She was able to walk out of the hospital in 3 days, and within 8 weeks she was back at work. In addition, she was able to garden, ride her horse, and even dance without experiencing pain.

Two months later Sarah began experiencing pain in her right knee; she attributed this to a recent hiking trip. Again, she waited for the pain to go away on its own. After 2 weeks, she started noticing that she was constantly rubbing her back, particularly at the end of the day. Also, she was waking up in the middle of the night with painful back spasms. Her anxiety about having another herniated disc created more sleep disturbances. She went back to the neurosurgeon, who found nothing abnormal upon examination and recommended waiting a few more weeks to see whether the pain would improve. But it increased, and Sarah stopped doing anything requiring physical effort.

Once again she returned to the neurosurgeon, who performed magnetic resonance imaging (MRI); this revealed nothing abnormal, except for some increased scar tissue around the previous surgical (laminectomy) site. Because the scar tissue did not appear to press on the nerve roots, her pain would not be helped by an operation. The surgeon then asked whether Sarah had been under any stress lately. He recommended that she keep busy with her life and suggested that the problem would resolve itself in time. Sarah left his office in a daze. By the time she got home, her imagination was running wild. "I'm in pain. Why can't they find something? What if they missed something important?" Sarah thought about her aunt, who had had back pain and was told nothing was wrong; the aunt eventually died of cancer.

Sarah felt terrified and desperate. She could no longer do normal things around the house. Vacuuming was agonizing. Standing or sitting for any extended time was painful. Her patience with her students was becoming short, and she began to miss days at work. She was generally too tired to socialize; even when she did, she felt as though she was always complaining. After a period of time, her friends stopped calling. She felt exhausted, alone, defective, miserable, and unlovable. She no longer had control over her body. The pain was controlling her now.

One day Sarah decided she should be able to do what she needed to do in spite of the pain. She was tough; all she needed to do was push through her daily activities. She cleaned the house, taught her classes, and took a dozen aspirin that day to help keep the pain down. The next morning, she couldn't get out of bed.

Sarah then went to another surgeon, who ordered a myelogram. The test revealed no herniated disc, but the surgeon suggested that stabilizing the spine by a fusion would give her relief. Sarah was so desperate that she had the operation. But it didn't work, and the pain just continued. She became even more depressed. By now she was unable to work. Her disability insurance supplied some sustenance, but her income certainly was not the same as when she was working. Furthermore, the disability insurance representatives were harassing her with paperwork, which necessitated more trips to the various doctors to fill out the forms. The office staff members made her feel like a pest. The doctors never filled out the paperwork on time, and she always panicked at the end of the month if the check was late.

Sarah's family doctor told her to learn to live with her pain and referred her to a psychologist, who determined that her response to pain was normal. She agreed, but she wanted answers on how to take her pain away. More than anything else, she wanted to know why she was in so much pain.

If this story feels familiar to you, you are not alone. Many people with chronic pain have experienced similar frustrations. You may have even been able to relate to Sarah's feelings about her pain. Were you able to identify the characteristics of acute versus chronic pain in this story?

Let's examine chronic pain once again. Chronic pain can be present either following an injury (as in Sarah's case) or without a specific injury. For example, in disorders such as fibromyalgia (see Appendix A), people can experience waxing and waning of joint and muscle aches, fatigue, and insomnia. Yet there may be no specific injury to explain the pain. The diagnosis is made by eliminating other disorders, such as rheumatoid arthritis or lupus. There is no specific treatment for fibromyalgia—all we can do is treat the insomnia and body aches. However, the experience of pain is just as complex and consuming as one stemming from a specific injury.

Whether your pain has a clear explanation or not, the persistence of your symptoms probably has multiple consequences. In fact, feelings of isolation and despair at the loss of physical and social activities may have become symptoms in their own right. Without effective ways of responding (called coping skills), you are likely to feel helpless and hopeless. In this program, you'll learn how to strengthen your present coping skills as well as develop new ones.

Remember that your experiences are real and normal and that your responses are understandable. At the same time, it is possible to do better and feel better.

The Processes Involved in Acute and Chronic Pain

Let's take a closer look at how acute and chronic pain is created. I'll describe the processes involved and then explain the rationale for treatment.

The pain response pathway is a two-way street. Sensory messages move into the spinal cord and up to the brain; signals then come back from the brain to the spinal cord and out through motor nerves. Motor nerves and sensory nerves are two major types of peripheral nerves. Motor nerves are like electrical wires that connect muscles to their power source, the brain and spinal cord. The fast motor reflexes enable us to remove our body out of harm's way. For example, they make us recoil after touching a hot iron. They can also protect the site of an injury by inducing muscle spasms to splint the injured area. Sensory nerves are more like thermostats that send a signal to the furnace when the room temperature rises or falls. There are a variety of sensory nerves, and some of them carry pain messages.

The Role of Sensory Nerves in Pain

Under normal circumstances, the sensory nerves that carry pain messages sit quietly until an event stimulates them into action. Pain receptors are located all over the body in the skin, muscles, joints, and internal organs. They respond to events such as damaging extremes of heat and cold, accidental or surgical trauma or chemical messengers (substance P, bradykinin, cytokines) released during injury and inflammation or extreme stretching. Whatever the original cause of the alarm, the pain nerves serve as the common pathway for pain information entering the spinal cord.

There are at least two types of sensory nerve fibers thought to carry the majority of pain messages to the spinal cord: "A-delta fibers" and "C fibers." These nerves carry messages at different speeds.

A common experience may help you to understand this process. You hit the so-called funny bone in your elbow (actually your ulnar nerve). The likely first sensation is a sharp, tingling pain right where you hit the elbow. This pain sensation probably results from the activity of the A-delta nerve fibers. They carry their electrical message to the spinal cord at approximately 40 miles an hour. Usually there is a second sensation, more like a vague, poorly localized ache, that spreads slowly up and down the inside of your arm. This is thought to result from the activity of C fibers, which carry their electrical message at approximately 3 miles per hour to the spinal cord. This difference in rate of speed contributes to the symphony of pain sensation at the time of an injury.

There are other types of sensory nerves that carry sensations besides pain. For example, after you hit your elbow, you automatically start to rub the area. This can work to soothe the painful area because it stimulates nerves that carry messages at approximately 180 to 200 miles per hour. These nerves, called A-beta fibers, carry pressure and touch messages. They race to the spinal cord to compete for attention with the incoming pain messages carried by the C fibers (3 miles per hour) and A-delta fibers (40 miles per hour).

Not all sensations are created equal, and you can make use of this fact for pain relief. You may have already found it helpful to apply massage, heat (including ultrasound), or ice to the painful area and/or to use transcutaneous electrical nerve stimulation (TENS) or acupuncture. Because of the way the nervous system works, these techniques can temporarily alter or decrease the pain message, depending on the intensity of the pain signal.

The Role of the Spinal Cord in Pain

Once a pain message has made it to the spinal cord as an electrical impulse, a very complicated system acts to send, modify, or cancel the message to the brain. In the spinal cord, the receiving nerve cells choose from among the messages received before they send the message forward to the brain. The choice is based on how loud the message is (the strength and duration), how many times the same message is received (repetition), and the overall number of other competing messages being received. The receiving nerve cells can be influenced by chemicals that can make the message louder (such as substance P and glutamate—targets of new pain research). They can also be influenced by dampening messages sent downstream from the brain. Substances such as serotonin, noradrenaline, and endorphin (*endo* = endogenous, *orphin* = morphine, the body's own natural pain reliever) are involved in reducing or blocking the pain signal. We call this downward alteration in the pain signal "modulation." The modulation process helps determine just how much of the pain message gets sent to the brain to be acted upon, both physically and emotionally. Thus rubbing the painful area or having a supportive spouse or friend present during labor and delivery may alter the pain experience.

The Role of the Brain in Pain

Once a pain signal makes its way to the brain, the brain responds to the strength, repetition, and duration of the pain message. As we saw above, the brain can fire impulses down the spinal cord to modulate the pain signal. Through connections with the cerebral cortex and limbic system (the "seat" of emotions), the pain message becomes a conscious and emotional experience. We do not see where all the electrical and chemical signals go, but we see the grimacing, limping, rubbing, and moaning that are the results of pain reaching awareness. The brain gives meaning to the pain message, and from meaning springs the emotional response, the source of suffering. But the brain is also the source of our ability to learn and to cope.

What Happens in Chronic Pain?

We know that long-lasting (chronic) pain often comes with diseases that involve long-term inflammation such as rheumatoid arthritis, myositis (muscle inflammation), lupus arthritis, and osteoarthritis. In these cases, the diseases continually set off the acute (normal) pain pathways through chronic inflammation. When such diseases come under remission or are modified, the pain is generally modified as well.

Why does pain persist in some people and not others after an injury or "successful" surgery? We are beginning to understand that there are multiple mechanisms involved. The only consistent predictor of developing chronic pain after an injury has been whether a person reported an unusually high level of pain during the acute pain episode. Is this genetic, environmental, or a response to a damaged pain system? We don't know.

We know from animal and human research that damaged pain nerves can start firing spontaneously. They become irritable and noisy, producing pain long after the original harm is done. For example, there are diseases that become associated with chronic pain because of pain-nerve damage occurring as a result of the disease process, such as in diabetes, HIV infection, and post-shingles neuropathy. Nerves can also be damaged by some therapies, as in radiation and chemotherapy-related neuritis (nerve inflammation). Scar tissue that develops during healing may constrict or pinch nerves and damage them.

Damage to pain nerves may be associated with experiencing pain even after light touch; spontaneous sensations of burning, pins and needles; or itching. The pain may be found to spread beyond the original site of injury to involve the whole arm or leg. In some individuals with complex regional pain syndrome (CRPS), Type 1 (see Appendix A), other nerve types are recruited into the pain process, with abnormal sweating, swelling, and blood vessel constriction or abnormal muscle movements in the affected limb. Such symptoms reflect multiple processes occurring in both the peripheral nerves and the central nervous system.

Indeed, recent research into pain mechanisms has shown that remarkable events occur when the spinal cord and brain are bombarded with persistent, high levels of pain. Changes take place that magnify, spread, and perpetuate pain. These changes take place in areas of the spinal cord where pain is usually processed and modified. This may cause the nerves to lose their ability to respond to the normal checks and balances that serve to dampen or alter the pain. Eventually the spinal cord nerves, and the brain centers they serve, may begin to perpetuate the pain signal independently long after the original injury has healed.

While the complexity may seem overwhelming, this increased level of understanding of what might be causing chronic pain should give hope for future treatments, if not cures. Genetic or stem cell research may provide the potential for predicting and eventually treating those individuals who develop chronic pain. Today there are many ways you can triumph over pain by understanding the pain process and doing your part to keep the pain at a stable level. This program will show you how.

The Chapter So Far

The first part of this chapter has done the following:

- Described the different parts of the normal pain pathway.
- Described the role of these parts—peripheral nerves, spinal cord, and brain—in chronic pain.
- Presented the current thinking about why chronic pain occurs.

With this groundwork laid, we next look more closely at ways that pain can be reduced by treating components of the pain process: inflammation, muscle spasm, nerve irritability, mood, and behavior. We will also look at existing treatments for reducing, *not curing*, chronic pain.

Treatments for Reducing Chronic Pain

There isn't enough scientific research on many pain treatments to know with certainty whether they help. Pain is a subjective, personal experience and research requires a standard definition of what improvement looks like. Even so, in some areas recommendations can be made based on solid scientific evidence that a treatment is effective—at reducing (not curing) pain. For each treatment discussed below, I note if there is enough research evidence to support a recommendation.

These evidence-based treatment recommendations are made by researchers and clinicians who have systematically evaluated all the research on that treatment. The conclusions they reach on the strength of the evidence are then offered as treatment guidelines. The National Guideline Clearinghouse (*www.guideline.gov*) serves as a global resource for all the guidelines that have been produced in this manner. The guideline for using pain medicine for osteoarthritis reproduced in Appendix D is one example of an evidence-based synthesis. Its aim is to assist the consumer in making an informed decision where there is no one absolutely correct answer. These resources are invaluable when available.

Don't be too disappointed when adequate research is not available for a particular medication or intervention. This is the case with many pain therapies. We are left to carefully monitor the effects of any treatment or intervention the best way we can and to be wary of promises of miracle cures or of no side effects until the evidence is in.

Reducing Inflammation

In chronic pain conditions such as rheumatoid arthritis, the immune process has gone haywire, allowing abnormal inflammation to occur. Instead of contributing to a normal healing process, it becomes an unregulated source of destruction. Other chronic pain syndromes associated with inflammation are lupus arthritis, ankylosing spondylitis, and possibly osteoarthritis. We do not know the extent of inflammation in other chronic pain conditions. Microinflammation may be involved, so a trial of anti-inflammatory agents may prove helpful. However, choosing among the many anti-inflammatory medications has become increasingly complex due to issues of safety and cost.

Inflammation is often treated with over-the-counter medications such as aspirin or naproxen. These nonsteroidal anti-inflammatory drugs (NSAIDs) block the effect of some of the chemicals released by damaged cells. They can help with mild to moderate pain but they can also have harmful side effects. The prescription NSAIDs known as COX-2 inhibitors can increase risk for heart attack. One such drug, Vioxx®, was withdrawn from the market. Another, Celebrex®, is still available. Possible side effects of NSAIDs include the following:

- Longer bleeding times
- Stomach irritation and bleeding
- Colitis (inflammation of the colon)
- "Rebound pain"—for example, the perpetuation of headache pain as a result of continuous use of analgesic medication
- Ankle swelling
- Kidney damage
- Increased risk of a heart attack

Increased risk of heart attack is also possible with older drugs such as ibuprofen (Motrin®, Advil®) at doses of 800 mg three times a day and diclofenac (Voltaren®) at 75 mg twice a day. Naproxen (Naprosyn®) does not appear to increase heart attack risk but, like all NSAIDs, it can still contribute to abdominal bleeding, particularly in older people. If you use aspirin for heart attack or stroke prevention, talk with your medical doctor about which anti-inflammatory you should be taking in addition. As mentioned above, Appendix D offers a helpful consumer guide to anti-inflammatory medications, "Choosing Pain Medicine for Osteoarthritis." This guide, as well as other useful information for consumers, is also available from *www.effectivehealthcare.ahrq.gov*. Take along a copy of the guide when you talk to your physician.

More severe inflammation may also be treated with medications that block the immune system response. For example, the immunosuppressant drug methotrexate, the tumor necrosis factor inhibitor Enbrel®, and the corticosteroid prednisone may be used in rheumatoid arthritis, Crohn's disease, or lupus arthritis. These medications decrease disease-producing inflammation and tissue destruction. They too have many potentially harmful side effects and should be used under careful medical supervision.

Finally, Tylenol® or acetaminophen can be effective for mild to moderate pain.

Many stronger opioid pain medications also include acetaminophen. It may have an action in the brain as well as in the periphery. It is not for inflammation treatment. It can be toxic to the liver if large quantities are taken—doses greater than 3,000 to 4,000 mg per day. If you use it over the long term, even at acceptable doses, then your doctor should monitor you with periodic liver and kidney function tests. Note: it is easier than you may think to take acetaminophen in large quantities because it is included in so many cold, flu, allergy, and pain preparations. It is important to read the labels to see how much additional acetaminophen you are getting if you take it regularly.

Take a moment to answer the following questions:

What anti-inflammatory medications do you use, if any? Include any over-the-counter brands. _____

_____

What possible side effects have you experienced? _____

_____

If you use these medications daily, has your kidney and liver function or blood count been tested in the past year? _____ If not, you should discuss this with your doctor.

Reducing Muscle Spasms

Some pain conditions are marked by muscle spasms. The muscles may become tight as a result of nerve irritation, reflexive guarding of a painful area, or generalized tension. Therefore, muscle relaxants (e.g., Norflex®, Flexeril®) are often prescribed to relax or loosen the muscles.

Scientists think these medications work primarily on the brain, except for Valium®, which also has a direct effect on skeletal muscles. With many of these medications, it is unclear how much of the relaxation is due to the brain's "relaxing" and how much is due to the skeletal muscles' relaxing. People often feel drowsy or sedated or have poor concentration when taking muscle relaxants because of their effect on the brain. Taking such medication long term is probably not helpful unless your problem is associated with spasticity (jerky, spastic movements), and even then medications like baclofen or tizanidine may be more helpful.

Researchers have looked at the evidence on use of muscle relaxants. They found that the benefits tend to outweigh the harm when they are used for limited treatment of chronic pain flare-ups and acute low back pain.

Other methods used to release muscle tension and reduce spasm include the following:

- Muscle massage (effect on chronic low back pain not supported by research to date)
- Acupuncture (research supports benefits for low back pain)

- Application of heat or ice
- Injection of tender areas of muscle or soft tissue called "trigger points" (effect on low back pain not supported by research)
- Relaxation response techniques
- Body awareness training
- Gentle stretching

The last three techniques will be addressed in detail in the next two chapters. Research shows all are likely to help chronic low back pain when part of an intensive multidisciplinary program.

Take a moment to answer the following questions:

Are you taking muscle relaxants? ____ If so, what are they? _____

_____

What possible side effects have you experienced? _____

_____

What other things have you done to release muscle tension? _____

_____

Reducing Pain Nerve Irritability

Perhaps the most exciting developments in chronic pain treatment come from the study of brain and spinal cord pain pathways. New techniques such as positron emission tomography (PET) and functional magnetic resonance imaging (fMRI) allow scientists to look at the brain in action. They have been able to study how and where the pain message is processed in the brain. New ideas for altering the pain system's response are emerging, including new uses for older medications. For example, some anti-seizure medications as well as some antidepressants have been found to have separate positive effects on nerve and brain pain pathways. I say more about these below.

In addition, researchers are trying to create opioids without the addiction side effect and to find more convenient and targeted medication delivery methods. Genetic explorations have begun but will most likely take a decade or more to translate into treatment options. The Internet Resources section at the back of the book lists websites for active clinical trials. These can tell you what chronic pain medications and interventions are now being tested. In some cases, you can volunteer to participate if you wish.

Medications may be used to alter pain nerve irritability in the body (peripheral nerves) and in the central nervous system (spinal cord and brain). Many of these medications are used "off label"; that is, the Food and Drug Administration (FDA) originally approved them for use in diseases or syndromes other than chronic pain. Because the actual way most drugs work is not completely understood, clinicians are given some flexibility to use medications off label if there is a sound rationale for trying them. Drugs with off-label use for chronic pain include tricyclic antidepressants, such as amitriptyline (Elavil®), imipramine, and nortriptyline. Baclofen, a muscle relaxant, is used by some for diabetic neuropathy. Good research evidence now exists that amitriptyline helps chronic pain, but it is still not approved by the FDA for that purpose.

Several anti-seizure medications have received FDA approval for use in neuropathies. Gabapentin (Neurontin®) is approved for neuropathic pain and post-shingles neuropathy, carbamazepine (Tegretol®) for trigeminal (facial sensory nerve) pain, clonazepam (Klonopin®) for neuralgia, and pregabalin (Lyrica®) for diabetic neuropathy, post-shingles neuropathy, and fibromyalgia. Tiagabine (Gabitril®) and phenytoin (Dilantin®) are used off label for pain but are not first choices because of lack of evidence that they are effective.

Zostrix® is an ointment made from the active ingredient in red chili peppers (capsaicin). It is used for pain associated with diabetes, shingles, osteoarthritis, and rheumatoid arthritis. A patch saturated with 5% lidocaine (Lidoderm®) can be applied directly to the skin of those suffering from post-shingles pain.

Nerve blocks with Novocain®-like substances and steroids have been injected in an attempt to quiet the firing of irritable nerves. Reviews of studies of epidural steroids and other local injections for low back pain have not yet demonstrated effectiveness, and facet joint injections are considered ineffective and possibly harmful.

Electrical stimulation of the peripheral nerves, spinal cord, and brain to override the pain messages may be used to reduce chronic pain. There may be short-term positive benefits of electrical stimulation in failed back surgery syndrome and complex regional pain syndromes, but more studies have been recommended.

Finally, sumatriptan (Imitrex®) and numerous other triptan-like medications are FDA-approved for treatment of migraine and cluster headaches. These medications are thought to work by activating serotonin receptors in the blood vessels. This causes narrowing of the blood vessels in the head and brain that contribute to the headache syndromes.

With continuing research to help us understand what makes pain chronic, new medications and therapies will become available. In the next decade, long-acting local anesthetics may be available to block sensory nerves for months instead of minutes. Drugs will be developed to disarm the mechanisms in the central nervous system that serve to wind up and magnify pain, and make it persist. There will be a new understanding of ways to prevent pain from becoming chronic. It is a worldwide effort.

Take a moment to answer the following questions about your treatment:

Are you taking medications to quiet nerve irritability? _____ If so, what are they? _____

_____

What are the possible side effects? _____

_____

What other treatments have you tried to quiet the irritable nerves? _____

_____

Helping the Brain Help You

As mentioned before, the brain can both raise and lower the loudness of pain messages. A great many internal and external events influence which direction the brain goes in. Insomnia, depression, anxiety, and alcohol dependence hurt the ability of the brain to function well. They can make the pain experience worse; preventing or reversing them can do the opposite.

Help for Insomnia

Insomnia or poor sleep quality can make the experience of pain more difficult. We need sleep for good health, but just how sleep refreshes and repairs the body remains largely unknown. Many problems, including pain, can be made worse by poor sleep.

People in pain who have sleep disorders are often treated with low doses of tricyclic antidepressants such as Elavil® (amitriptyline) or imipramine. These medications help with sleep because they tend to produce drowsiness, although some people need to take them up to 4 hours before bedtime. In very low dosages these medications also appear to alter pain sensitivity in some disorders. The exact way they do this is unknown, but some change in norepinephrine and/or serotonin levels in the brain or spinal cord has been suggested. Remember that serotonin is one of the pain-dampening chemicals in the brain and spinal cord mentioned earlier. In addition, serotonin is believed to play a role in depression. This may be why the older tricyclic antidepressants and the newer ones like duloxetine (Cymbalta®) can improve both depression and some chronic pain syndromes.

There are other ways you can help yourself sleep better. Going to bed and waking up at the same time every day is important. If naps are necessary, sleep only for 30–45 minutes. Take a hot shower or bath about 2 hours before bedtime; this will raise your body temperature, and the cooling down afterward can help trigger sleep. A small carbohydrate snack before bed can also induce sleep. If you've been trying to fall asleep (or go back to sleep) for more than 30 minutes, get up and do something until you feel sleepy again. Often people become anxious as they lie in bed with their eyes wide open. Continuing to struggle with sleep simply makes it less likely. The relaxation response techniques described in the next chapter are particularly helpful if you practice them before you go to bed or if you wake up during the night.

If your insomnia is associated with snoring, sleep apnea (periods of not breathing while asleep), or excessive daytime drowsiness, it may be helpful to make an appointment with a sleep disorders clinic.

Help for Depression and Anxiety

Many people with chronic pain experience depression and anxiety, and these feelings can change the pain experience for the worse. People who experience significant depression in addition to pain usually feel helpless and powerless. Anxiety makes people with pain even more frightened by their loss of control, and they have a heightened level of tension. It is important to treat these conditions. Bringing disabling depression and anxiety (such as panic attacks) under control may require medication. There is evidence that the antidepressant duloxetine (Cymbalta®) can help in the pain syndrome fibromyalgia and in diabetic neuropathy, for which it is approved by the FDA. Short-acting benzodiazepines, such as Xanax® and Ativan®, are suited for short-term use for brief bouts of anxiety. However, longer-term use can have negative results without careful evaluation and a comprehensive treatment plan that includes non-drug treatment as well. I say more about coping with depression and anxiety in Chapters 5 and 6.

Reducing Use of Alcohol

Alcohol, an old remedy for acute pain, may temporarily change pain perception, but it does little to help with long-term coping, because nothing really changes. Alcoholism can be an additional complication of self-medicating pain with alcohol. In some cases, alcohol consumption before bedtime can actually disrupt sleep. Moreover, in certain people (particularly those prone to headaches or fibromyalgia), alcohol use can increase pain. A source of empty calories with no nutritional value, alcohol can contribute to weight gain. You will have the opportunity to explore how alcohol affects your pain in Chapter 7.

Take a moment to answer the following questions:

Do you have a drink from time to time to relieve your pain? _____

Have you ever felt you should cut down on your drinking? _____

Have people annoyed you by criticizing your drinking? _____

Have you ever felt bad or guilty about your drinking? _____

Have you ever had a drink first thing in the morning (an "eye opener") to steady your nerves or to get rid of a hangover? _____

If you have more than two "yes" answers, there is a high likelihood that you have a problem with alcohol. Seek help from your doctor, therapist, or someone else you trust. Talk to them about it. Chronic pain is bad enough—excessive alcohol use could harm you even more.

Using Narcotics (Opioids) in Chronic Pain

Opioid is the more accurate name for opium-like medicines such as morphine, Percocet®, and Vicodin®. Chronic pain does not respond to opioids in the same way that acute or cancer pain responds. This may be due to the different processes, discussed earlier, that create chronic pain. My colleagues and I do not recommend the use of opioids *instead of* taking an active role in managing chronic pain; however, opioids can have their place in helping some people reach their goals of living more fully and functioning better.

The goal of opioid treatment in chronic pain is not to be *pain free*, because that doesn't happen; the goal is to have more tolerable pain so that you can do more. The American Pain Society and the American Academy of Pain Medicine (organizations of professional pain specialists) both endorse the careful use of opioids in chronic pain when the other treatments we have already reviewed fail to give adequate pain control. People with no history of drug abuse have few problems when one physician (usually the patient's primary care physician) prescribes a constant dose of opioids taken on a regular schedule or under specific circumstances like starting a new exercise regime or traveling.

There are multiple preparations of opioids. Long-acting, time-released opioids are available for morphine, oxycodone, and fentanyl and tend to provide a constant blood level of medication. They are thought to contribute to more constant levels of pain relief. Methadone is an inexpensive, long-acting opioid alternative to the time-released opioids. CAUTION: There have been an increasing number of deaths due to using and misusing methadone and other long-acting, time-released opioids. Recent evidence suggests that methadone may be associated with rare but fatal arrhythmias (irregular heartbeats). In addition, the slow metabolism of methadone mandates that careful increases in dosing be made over many days to weeks. Avoid mixing of methadone with other opioids, particularly in the early period of dose adjustments. You can die if you add long-acting opioid preparations too quickly or increase the dosing above what has been prescribed.

One unusual medication, not classified as a narcotic or controlled substance, is tramadol, which resembles both morphine and tricyclic antidepressants. It binds weakly to morphine receptors and acts like amitriptyline in the central nervous system. Because it binds so weakly to the mu (morphine) receptor it is thought to be less addictive. It has been used with some success in patients looking for relief from their physical pain.

It is important that you discuss any side effects (nausea, constipation, drowsiness) of opioid treatment with your health care professional. These side effects can be treated effectively—and they should be—if the opioid is making a significant difference in pain control and function. The goal of opioid therapy is better pain control in order to allow you to do more. What activities are being stopped by your high pain level? Make a list. For example, is it exercise, shopping, sitting at the computer, going to the theater, volunteering, or all of the above? Careful pacing of activities and setting realistic goals will help you be more successful.

If you use a prescribed opioid, you have responsibilities. You should take the opioid only as directed, receive the opioid from one physician and one pharmacy, and report side effects promptly. Do not stop the drug abruptly or you risk having withdrawal symptoms. You should also use caution in the first few weeks of dose adjustments, because you may have difficulty thinking and using good judgment, and have a slower reaction time. When using an opioid you are also responsible for using other pain management skills such as those described in this book. Those skills reduce the amount of opioid you need. You will have less pain overall and need less opioid if you can attend to the other symptoms associated with chronic pain, such as insomnia, anxiety, muscle tension, and fatigue. Often opioids are misused in chronic pain because people lack the skills to cope with pain in any other way. Problems may develop when pain medications are taken to "relax," to induce sleep, to decrease the fear of anticipated pain increases, to reduce stress-based symptoms, or to alleviate frustration. These purposes are better served by using pain management techniques such as those described in the chapters that follow.

Opioids are addictive in some people. An addiction is more likely if you or a biologically related family member has a history of alcoholism or substance abuse, but you may be predisposed and not know it. Addiction is a complicated disorder that may be genetically determined but has a strong environmental component to its development as well. It is defined as an obsessive use of a substance (opioids, alcohol, even food) that results in physical, psychological, or social harm to the user and continues in spite of this harm.

The risk of addiction with opioids prescribed for chronic pain of uncertain cause poses challenges for both doctors and patients. I see no resolution to the question of effectiveness in chronic pain syndromes until we have more biological knowledge about addiction and chronic pain. In the interim, it's best to be evaluated and treated by a physician with chronic pain treatment experience before opioids are prescribed long term.

If you take opioids on a daily basis and anticipate any surgery, you will most likely need additional opioids for postsurgical pain control. After surgery you will need your daily dose of opioids plus as much as two to three times more than a person who is not taking opioids daily. Many doctors and nurses are not aware of this, so before surgery it is important for you to discuss the postoperative pain treatment with the anesthesiologist or surgeon who will be working with you. Likewise, should you have a new painful injury or condition, such as a bone fracture or kidney stones, you will also need additional opioids. These increases in opioids should not be required for more than the average recovery period.

There are patients whose pain does not respond to opioids. They find that the pain does not really change that much on or off the medication. They may even feel better once the opioid is tapered and stopped. We don't know the long-term effects of opioid treatment for chronic pain, although sexual dysfunction and impotence have been described in men. In spite of this, opioids help some people. A pain specialist can help you decide what is best for you.

Take a moment to answer the following questions:

Are you taking antidepressants for depression and/or anxiety? _____

_____

Are you taking opioids? _____

_____

What treatments do you use for side effects? _____

_____

Are you using any other medications for pain management that haven't been mentioned here? If so what are they? _____

_____

Do you understand why these medications have been recommended? _____ If not, where can you get this information? _____

_____

Make a Medication List—It Can Save Your Life!

Most people with chronic pain take medication, and it is important for you to know what you are taking, what it's for, and if it's working. Because a treatment can work for one person and not another it is very important to be able to report your experience with each treatment. Keeping your pain diary will help you do this. Keeping a list of your medications will also help—and it's more important. It can save your life!

Making a medication list is one of the exploration tasks at the end of this chapter but it's so important I want to mention it here as well. I urge you to complete it, carry it with you at all times, and keep it updated. Put *all* of your medications on the list, including over-the-counter and herbal medications and vitamins. This is particularly critical for individuals who take more than five medications per day. The current health care system is fragmented. Until we have a better way for prescription drug information to reach all those who give you care you will be safer if you can give your health care providers an accurate medication list.

The Meanings of Pain

Despite what we do know about pain, the fact remains that we are not able to take away chronic pain for the millions who suffer with it, but the suffering is optional.

Cultural Influences on Attitudes toward Pain

The way pain is treated in the Western hemisphere is strongly influenced by Western culture, and a booming pharmacological industry has had a sweeping effect on our attitudes toward pain treatment. The emphasis is on "quick fixes" and the use of medications for all our problems. There is much less emphasis on what patients can do for themselves to make their lives healthier and happier. Medicine does not have all the answers. The erroneous impression that it does is pervasive. David Morris comments on this in his book *The Culture of Pain*:

> Today our culture has willingly, almost gratefully, handed over to medicine the job of explaining pain. This development, accelerating with the prestige of science over the last several centuries, has brought with it consequences that remain almost completely unanalyzed. . . . Although almost all eras and cultures have employed doctors, never before in human history has the explanation of pain fallen so completely to medicine. (p. 19)

There is no simple explanation for pain, nor is there a good effective drug for each of the troubles we might experience. We can't wait for the definitive answers; we must have some way to manage symptoms now in spite of our incomplete knowledge, and solutions shouldn't be limited to drugs or medical procedures. However, many people don't realize that "medicine knows all" is only a cultural expectation, not a fact. They have not had the opportunity to explore the various influences on their pain experiences. This book and the program it describes will help you explore the multiple meanings of pain. It will help you see that adopting different attitudes toward pain is possible and can be very helpful.

Exercise: Exploring the Meanings of Pain

Here's a helpful exercise to explore how your pain has affected your activities, physical responses, thoughts, and feelings. Don't be surprised or alarmed if your responses to these questions cause you sadness, anger, or anxiety. This exercise will help you start to assess the full cost of your pain experience. It will also help you to begin to recognize ineffective ways of coping, so that you can replace them with more effective ones from the chapters to come.

1. How has your pain affected how you work, play, and perform other activities? _____

_____

_____

_____

_____

_____

_____

2. Besides the pain, what other physical symptoms do you experience (for example, insomnia, fatigue, etc.)? _____

_____

_____

_____

_____

_____

_____

3. What are your thoughts and feelings in response to your pain experience? _____

_____

_____

_____

_____

_____

_____

4. What does being in pain mean to you?

_____

_____

_____

_____

_____

_____

Please do the above exercise before continuing. It will help you understand what follows.

When I have patients do this exercise, the blackboard is filled with the real consequences of their daily pain. Samples of these responses are given in the table on the next page. It is obvious from looking at the list that people with chronic pain are very courageous to continue with their lives in spite of their suffering. For most, all aspects of their lives have been affected, and though it has been difficult, they have done the best they can. What becomes striking during the discussion that follows the exercise, however, is that for most of these people only their *physical* pain has been the focus of their medical treatment. The other parts of their pain experience—emotions, thoughts, and behaviors—have largely been ignored.

Activities decreased or stopped	Physical symptoms	Feelings and thoughts
Work	Fatigue	Anger
Pleasure (hobbies, movies)	Sweating	Depression
Household chores	Weight gain/loss	Anxiety
Sex	Headaches	Fear
Socializing	Decreased concentration	Guilt
Exercise	Palpitations (increased heart rate)	Frustration
Family activities		Out of control
Sports	Shortness of breath	Can't do what I used to
	Decreased memory	Hopeless/helpless
	Diarrhea	No one understands
	Muscle tension	"Why me?"
	Insomnia	"When will this go away?"
	Constipation	"I can't go on."
	Body aches	Failure
		Unlovable
		Ugly
		Denial

The False Division of Mind and Body

Much of the suffering you have identified in the previous exercise arises out of a common misunderstanding in Western culture that there is a division between mind and body. This division is reinforced daily. Medical doctors take care of our bodies, and psychologists or psychiatrists take care of our minds. Our hearts are looked after by heart specialists, our stomachs by stomach specialists, and so on. In the last 20 years there has been a growing discontent with the fragmentation of our bodies and minds. Such terms as "behavioral medicine" and "holistic medicine" have been used to describe the integration of mind and body in medical practice.

The division between mind and body is a false one. Nowhere is that falseness more obvious than in dealing with chronic pain. The experience of pain is a coming together of many personal factors, such as the following:

- The pain signal
- Expectations of yourself and of others
- Self-esteem
- Ability to function
- Mood

- Hormones
- Genetics
- Previous traumas
- Injustices and beliefs
- Coping styles

It is not in your best interest to deny these influences on your pain or to act as if nothing is wrong. If you deny the pain, push on, and regularly do things that increase the pain, you only make your condition worse. Even if the consequences aren't immediate (you can't get out of bed), they are cumulative (stress symptoms). Taking this path sets you up for endless frustration and loss of control.

However, pretending that nothing is wrong is not the same as making a conscious decision to act for a particular purpose knowing that increased discomfort will follow. For example, Mary wanted to take her granddaughter to the circus. She knew that sitting through the performance would increase her pain. She prepared herself with an extra cushion and sat in the back row so that she could stand periodically. Her pain did increase, but she was not upset because she felt it worth the effort, and her granddaughter was thrilled. The activity was her choice, and it was under her control.

The key is to ask, "Where do I have control?" If you can acknowledge your pain and make conscious decisions about your activities, you will not feel so victimized. As one patient said, "If I sit, I'm in pain. If I walk, I'm in pain. So I might as well walk and get somewhere." If the pain is part of your life, it is important to work with it; this is where you have the control.

You probably feel a fair amount of external pressure to act as if nothing is wrong and to ignore what you know to be necessary. You can change your attitude toward your pain, increase your activities safely, and have a life in addition to the pain. The rest of this book will help you do just that.

The misunderstandings that arise out of the separation of mind and body are not limited to people who actually experience chronic pain. Many physicians refuse to acknowledge that physical pain is associated with psychological suffering. This refusal gives rise to the "psychological illness" stigma. When people express sadness or anxiety about their pain, others often assume that these emotional symptoms are the *cause* of their pain. There is a tendency to label such people as "hysterics" or "hypochondriacs" or to dismiss the problem as "not real" (that is, not physical). Many individuals experience this stigma when their physicians cannot explain the physical cause of persistent pain.

Likewise, the failure to address psychological and social issues early in the course of pain treatment devalues these important aspects of the pain experience. Skills such as relaxation techniques are usually offered only *after* a patient has "failed" to respond to medications or nerve blocks. Until recently, primary care physicians received no formal training in forms of pain management other than the use of medications. While pain management is now included in physician training programs, it is limited to acute pain and a focus on physical symptoms. Mind–body approaches to pain management have been overlooked not because they are ineffective but because they remain unknown to the majority of those providing treatment. They are also not the quick fix that so many Americans demand.

So what is the problem? And whose problem is it, anyway? The problem is, of course, that you have pain, and it is not going away. In keeping with the philosophy of this program, I strongly recommend that you acknowledge the problem is yours, since you are the one in pain. If you hand it over to your physician, family, or society, you simply lose the opportunity to have some control over it.

Where Do You Go from Here?

In the following chapters, the physical symptoms that you have identified in the previous exercise are addressed through a series of skills and techniques aimed at reducing stress. These symptoms reveal the wear and tear on the body from prolonged pain and the failure to heed the mind–body, body–mind connection. Techniques such as the relaxation response, breath exercises, stretching, and body awareness exercises will help you nurture your body and counteract the stress symptoms.

You have also identified decreases in your physical and social activities, along with increased isolation. To address these symptoms, you will learn to monitor the way you pace yourself during activity, to interpret your pain sensations, and to add pleasurable activities and exercise to your regular routine.

You have also begun to identify negative, self-defeating thoughts and feelings. Cognitive therapy techniques will help you examine how this negative self-talk distorts what is really happening around you. You will learn how to be more realistic and self-empowering. Humor will be used to soften the hard work and the slow pace at which real change proceeds. Communication skills will encourage self-esteem and the assertiveness required to identify your needs. Improving your problem-solving abilities in regard to the challenges of pain will allow you to participate fully in society once again and to achieve the goals you set for yourself.

Summary

Pain

- Pain is a symptom that indicates harm to the body.

- Pain is a complex process that can be changed for better or worse by people's perceptions.

- There are two categories of pain:

—Acute pain is time-limited and its cause is usually known. Cancer can cause acute pain but its duration can be longer than other kinds of acute pain.

—Chronic pain is pain that lasts longer than 3 months. Its exact cause may not be known. Chronic pain can be the result of painful chronic diseases, nerve damage, or the loss of the normal checks and balances involved in modulating pain signals in the brain or spinal cord.

- The pain response pathway is a two-way street: Sensory nerves carry pain signals to the spinal cord and up to the brain. Modulation of the pain message takes place by downward impulses from the brain. Motor nerves carry motor reflexes from the spinal cord to the muscles.

Sensory Nerves

- Pain nerves are stimulated by extremes of hot or cold, trauma, or chemicals released during inflammation.

- Two types of sensory nerves carry pain messages to the spinal cord:
  - —A-delta fibers carry the pain messages at approximately 40 miles per hour.
  - —C fibers carry pain messages at approximately 3 miles per hour.

- Other sensory nerves carry pressure and touch. These are A-beta fibers, which travel at approximately 180 miles per hour. Some pain can be reduced by rubbing or applying pressure.

- Chronic pain may develop when there is a painful chronic disease, when an injured pain nerve is damaged and attempts to regenerate, or when there are changes in the pain nerve modulation system.

Inflammation

- Inflammation is a process that fights infection or cleans up and repairs tissue damage.

- When inflammation occurs, cells in the body release chemicals that signal the pain nerves, muscles, and blood vessels that damage control must begin.

Muscles

- Muscle spasm or tightness can guard a painful area. Nerve irritation and generalized tension can also lead to muscle spasm.

- Muscle relaxants are thought to work primarily in the brain to loosen the muscles, so they have side effects like drowsiness.

The Spinal Cord and Brain

- There is competition among the sensory nerve messages as they come into the spinal cord; not all pain messages get attention.
- Substances sent downstream from the brain can reduce or block pain signals.
- The brain gives meaning to the pain message.
- Poor brain function can make the pain experience worse.
- Sleep problems, depression, anxiety, and alcohol dependence can all lead to poor brain function and make the pain experience more difficult.

Treatments

- There is little evidence to support the effectiveness of many treatments used for chronic pain, but evidence-based treatment guidelines are starting to appear.
- Sometimes medications are effective in calming irritated nerves.
- Inflammation is treated with anti-inflammatory medications such as aspirin or naproxen. These drugs block the effects of some of the chemicals released during inflammation.
- Treatments to release muscle tension and prevent spasm include massage, acupuncture, heat or ice application, trigger point injections, relaxation response techniques, and body awareness training.
- Muscle relaxants are best used for limited treatment of short-term chronic pain flare-ups or acute low back pain.
- Following good sleep recommendations can be helpful. Medications are not recommended for long-term sleeping disorders.
- Treating depression and anxiety improves brain function and can reduce chronic pain.
- The use of alcohol does little to help with long-term coping, carries the risk of abuse, and can actually disrupt sleep and increase pain.
- The use of opioids should be decided on an individual basis with the treating physician.
- The goal of opioid treatment in chronic pain is to reduce disabling pain and increase activities.
- Opioids should not be the only treatment used in chronic pain.
- There are guidelines for using opioids in chronic pain.
- New treatment ideas are emerging as we learn more about the pain system and how it functions.

The Meanings of Pain

- The idea that medicine has all the answers for pain is only a cultural expectation, not a fact.
- Chronic pain has many meanings for everyone who suffers from it.
- The experience of pain involves both mind *and* body; many patients have suffered from the artificial division between mind and body.
- Physical pain is associated with psychological suffering.
- By acknowledging the pain and making conscious decisions about your activities, you will gain some control over it.

Exploration Tasks

1. Answer all the questions in this chapter on medication, and get information on each medication that you take from your pharmacist, *Physicians' Desk Reference*, or MedlinePlus (*www.nlm.nih.gov/medlineplus/druginformation.html*).

2. Safeguard yourself: make a medication list. Millions of people are harmed every year by medication errors. Good and well-intentioned people can make mistakes. One of the most important things you can do for yourself is to make a medication list, keep it updated, and carry it with you at all times. Every pill you put in your mouth should be documented on your list. There is a sample list at the end of this chapter and a blank copy at the end of the book. There are also multiple websites where you can store details on your medications and other essential medical information, such as your medical diagnoses, family doctor's and specialists' names, immunizations, and so forth. Many people visit multiple doctors, are hospitalized away from home or away from critical medical information, and may be taking multiple medications. When a chronic problem like pain is involved, an up-to-date medication list can be life saving. Typing "online personal medical records" into your search engine will allow you to explore online or off-line personal health record formats that might help organize your health history.

Supplementary Reading

The following books provide additional information on the pain process and on maintaining health:

Herbert Benson and Eileen Stuart, *The Wellness Book: The Comprehensive Guide to Maintaining Health and Treating Stress-Related Illness* (New York: Fireside, 1993).

Charles B. Berde, "Pain, Anxiety, Distress, and Suffering: Interrelated, But Not Interchangeable," *Journal of Pediatrics, 142,* 361–363, 2003.

Howard L. Fields, *Pain Mechanisms and Management, Second Edition* (New York: McGraw-Hill, 2001).

Gary W. Jay, *Chronic Pain* (Boca Raton, FL: CRC Press, 2007).

Mayo Clinic, *Mayo Clinic on Chronic Pain* (New York: Kensington, 1999).

David Morris, *The Culture of Pain* (Berkeley: University of California Press, 1991).

Robert Ornstein and David Sobel, *The Healing Brain* (Los Altos, CA: Malor Books, 1999).

R. C. Rinaldi, E. M. Steindler, B. B. Wilford, and D. Goodwin, "Clarification and Standardization of Substance Terminology," *Journal of the American Medical Association, 259,* 555–557, 1988.

Dennis C. Turk and Frits Winter, *The Pain Survival Guide: How to Reclaim Your Life* (Washington, DC: American Psychological Association, 2005).

Patrick Wall and Steven Rose (Eds.), *Pain: The Science of Suffering* (New York: Columbia University Press, 2000).

Carol Warfield and Zahid Bajwa, *Principles and Practice of Pain Medicine, Second Edition* (New York: McGraw-Hill, 2004).

Medication List

Name _____   List last updated _____

Medication	How is it prescribed?	Pill dose?	Total dose per day	What's it for?	Morning	Midday	Evening	Bedtime	Prescribed by	Over the counter? (Check if yes)
amitriptyline	2 pills at bedtime	10 mg	20 mg	nerve pain and sleep				10 pm	Dr. Smith	
naproxen sodium	2 pills 2X/day	220 mg	880 mg	inflammation	8 am		8 pm			✓

3
The Mind–Body Connection

*I had forgotten that my body was also a sanctuary, a
haven. . . . I felt it had betrayed me and tortured me for
so many years.*

The above comment was made by Mary, a program participant, about her pain experience after practicing the techniques that are described in this chapter.

Chronic Pain as a Form of Chronic Stress

As indicated in Chapter 2, the mind and body are really one. They never have been separate and never should have been viewed as separate. How you feel (happy, sad, angry) can influence and be influenced by your body's processes. For instance, you may have noticed that on a day when your pain is particularly bad, you have trouble concentrating or lose your appetite. You may have also noticed that when you are intensely focused on an activity (such as watching a football playoff or talking with your best friend), your pain, for that time, slips out of consciousness. Because this mind–body connection is so intimate, the experience of "stress"—defined here as the *perception* of a threat and the perception that you are not well prepared to cope with it—can lead to both physical and emotional symptoms.

Human beings have an automatic, biological response to the perception of threat or danger, called the "fight-or-flight response." Let's look at the following scenario:

> It is late at night and you are home alone. You wake up to the sound of a crash downstairs. Your heart starts to beat rapidly; your muscles tense up; you feel anxious and short of breath. You may not be aware of it, but the hair on the back of your neck is standing on end, your blood pressure is increasing, and the

pupils of your eyes are dilating. Blood is moving from your stomach to the skeletal muscles in preparation for their rapid movement out of harm's way. Your body is preparing to fight or flee.

The first thing you do is grab a flashlight and quietly make your way downstairs. Trembling, you listen for further sounds. As you reach the bottom of the stairs, you see that the "intruder" is your cat dashing away from a broken vase. Within minutes after the "danger" has passed, your physical state returns to normal and your fear passes.

The changes in your body that constitute the fight-or-flight response (increased heart and breath rate, increased blood pressure, changes in blood flow to muscles, etc.) are caused by the release of adrenaline and other hormones from the sympathetic nervous system. The effect is to put your body into temporary overdrive to meet the challenge of threat or danger. When you are constantly in this stressed state, however, your body can go beyond its capacity for reestablishing homeostasis (balance). Your body's abilities to restore itself to normal can be exhausted. This can contribute to numerous symptoms:

- Reduced immunity to disease
- Diarrhea and/or constipation
- Sleep disturbance
- Fatigue
- Headaches
- Poor concentration
- Shortness of breath
- Weight loss/gain
- Increased muscle tension
- Anxiety/depression

Chronic pain certainly fits the definition of a constant stressor. The physical stress that chronic pain places on your body results from a prolonged fight-or-flight response. How you perceive your ability to cope with the pain influences your stress level and your experience of pain. If you feel overwhelmed by your pain and do not take time to recover from the stress, you will most likely begin to experience stress-related symptoms like those listed above. This is why stress management techniques can be so helpful in chronic pain. Techniques that bring about the "relaxation response," as described next, will help you recover from the physical symptoms of stress; they will also prepare you to cope with pain more effectively.

The Relaxation Response (RR) Is Not the Same as Relaxing

The "relaxation response" (which will be abbreviated from here on in this book as "RR") was first described by Herbert Benson and his colleagues at Harvard Medical School in the early 1970s. The RR appears to play a role in quieting the body's responses to stress. However, unlike the fight-or-flight response, the RR is not automatic. Before it can be called on to counteract stress, certain mental techniques must be practiced.

After reviewing many religious and philosophical writings, Benson realized that for centuries humankind had been provided with instructions for bringing about this quieting reflex. He also realized that even though many techniques could bring about this natural bodily response, there were two simple steps common to them all:

1. Focusing one's mind on a repetitive phrase, word, breath, or action.

2. Adopting a passive attitude toward the thoughts that go through one's head.

From the extensive research done by Benson and others, we know that the regular practice of RR techniques makes it harder for the sympathetic nervous system to become aroused by daily hassles. In other words, it becomes less easy for the little frustrations of modern living to set off the fight-or-flight response, and when it is aroused it returns to normal more quickly. Thus, chronic stress symptoms are reduced or never develop. The physical effects of the RR can be divided into groups: immediate changes, which occur while a person is focusing on a repetitive word, phrase, breath, or action; and long-term changes, which happen after repeated practice for at least a month. The more immediate changes include a lowering of blood pressure, heart rate, breath rate, and oxygen consumption (which is a measure of metabolic rate). The long-term changes are thought to alter the body's response to adrenaline. People may report a decrease in anxiety and depression, as well as an improvement in their ability to cope with life stressors. These changes are present even when a person is not sitting quietly practicing an RR technique.

Many people confuse "feeling relaxed" with the RR. They are not the same unless what a person is doing to relax includes the two steps mentioned—focusing on something repetitive and having a passive attitude toward thoughts. In research using the RR, the controls—that is, the participants who will *not* be taught how to bring about the RR—are instructed instead to listen to music or read a book. Although under normal circumstances listening to music and reading a book may be relaxing, they do not bring about the RR.

To recap, the RR is a natural response of the body, but it needs to be trained and practiced. It is brought about by focusing the mind on a repeated word, phrase, breath, or action, and by a passive attitude toward interfering thoughts. It is not elicited by reading a book, listening to quiet music, sleeping, or hanging out. All of these may be relaxing, but they are not the same as bringing about the RR.

Using Breath to Relax and Focus Your Mind

The key to bringing about the RR is focused awareness. Your breathing can be the object of that focus. In addition, because normal breathing patterns can be disrupted by tension, stress, and pain, focusing on how you breathe may provide you with an additional method of relaxing.

There are two types of breathing: "chest breathing" and "diaphragmatic breathing" (better known as "abdominal breathing").

Chest Breathing

Many people, particularly women, are "chest breathers." That is, they suck in their abdomens and expand their chests with each in-breath. In Western culture, women are taught early in life that the "proper" posture is one in which the abdomen is flat at all times. This posture is difficult to maintain if a person breathes from the abdomen or "diaphragmatically," which requires the stomach to move in and out with each breath.

Many men and women also become chest breathers because of prolonged anxiety, stress, and tension. One reason for this may be that short, shallow breaths are characteristic of anxiety. Stress may also increase tension in the abdominal area, not allowing the diaphragm to contract completely or the abdominal wall to move out when taking an in-breath. Only the chest expands as a result, and the breath is not as deep.

Diaphragmatic Breathing

We all start out breathing diaphragmatically, with our abdomens rising and falling. Watch infants when they breathe: Their stomachs move with each breath. Over the years, many of us become chest breathers. Relearning to breathe diaphragmatically may feel strange at first, but with practice it can become second nature again.

The diaphragm is a thin dome of muscle that separates the chest cavity from the abdominal cavity. At the beginning of each in-breath, it contracts and the dome flattens out. Air is then pulled into the lungs, and the abdominal wall moves out. (Picture a balloon in the abdomen that fills with air on the in-breath.) When the diaphragm and the chest relax, the breath moves out and the abdomen flattens again. On the next in-breath, the process starts over. Because of this extra space for the lungs to fill, a diaphragmatic breath is a fuller and more complete breath than a chest breath.

For reasons that are still not altogether clear to physiologists, diaphragmatic breathing can bring about a feeling of calm and relaxation when it is purposefully done.

Breathing Exercises

It is recommended that you wear loose, comfortable clothing and that you find a quiet, relaxing place to engage in breathing exercises.

How Do You Breathe?

Before starting these exercises, you need to become aware of how you breathe.

1. Find a comfortable place and lie down on your back. If this is uncomfortable, try sitting in a chair.

2. Place one hand on your breastbone and one hand over your belly button.

3. Close your eyes and become aware of what is moving when you breathe in and out.

4. If your abdomen moves up and down (without your forcing it) with each breath, you are already breathing diaphragmatically. You can move on to the "Breath-Focusing Exercises" section later in this chapter. If your chest moves up and down with each breath, however, you need to practice breathing diaphragmatically. Go to the next section, "Diaphragmatic Breathing Exercises."

Diaphragmatic Breathing Exercises

Three diaphragmatic breathing exercises are provided here to help you train your awareness of what should be moving when you breathe diaphragmatically. If one position does not work out for you, try another. Once you are aware, you should be able to do diaphragmatic or abdominal breathing lying, sitting, or standing.

Sometimes when people focus on their breath, they tend to breathe too fast or too deeply. If you feel light-headed, dizzy, or anxious, you may be breathing too quickly or too deeply; just stop practicing for a moment and breathe normally until the symptoms pass. In addition, *do not do these exercises if these positions make your pain worse.*

Exercise 1

1. Find a comfortable place and lie on your stomach.

2. Lift your chest off the floor by bringing your elbows back against your side at the level of your shoulders. Then push off the floor with your forearms (like the Sphinx). This position will arch your back slightly.

3. Breathe normally. This will lock your chest so that when you breathe, the abdomen alone will move up and down.

Exercise 2

1. Sit in a chair and clasp your hands behind your head.

2. Point your elbows out to the side. Again, this serves to lock your chest so that you can feel the movement in your abdomen.

3. Breathe normally.

Exercise 3

1. Find a comfortable place and lie on your back.

2. Place your hands just below your belly button.

3. Close your eyes and imagine a balloon inside your abdomen.

4. Each time you breathe in, imagine the balloon filling with air.

5. Each time you breathe out, imagine the balloon collapsing.

Breath-Focusing Exercises

Now that you are aware of your breathing, you can start to practice breath focusing.

1. Make a tight fist and notice what happens to your breathing. Don't read on; just do it. Did you find that you held your breath or breathed in shallow, short spurts?

2. Now relax that fist.

3. Make a tight fist again, but this time continue to breathe normally. What happens to the tension in your fist? The tension should be reduced—and, in fact, should be difficult to maintain without a real effort.

Remember: *It's hard to maintain tension (stress, pain, anger, anxiety) and keep breathing.* This principle is used in Lamaze exercises for women in labor. The Lamaze technique focuses on breathing to release tension and increase control during the various stages of labor. Women are encouraged to use their breathing to control the pain. This same principle can be applied to your pain experience.

Observe how often you hold your breath when you anticipate pain or when you are experiencing pain. You can change this experience by breathing. When you experience pain (or increased tension, anger, anxiety, or stress), do the following:

1. Purposefully stop and pause.

2. Take a slow, deep breath from your diaphragm.

3. Focus on what you are doing and how you are feeling. What is the problem? What are your choices? Do you need to continue with a certain activity, or can you change what you are doing? Is the situation worth getting upset about at this moment?

As you will see, breath-focusing exercises can sometimes give you instant control, because they make you focus on the present moment. You may often be caught off guard by stressful events if you are busy worrying about the future, wishing you could change the past, or responding automatically without thinking at all. Focusing on the present moment allows you to consider more clearly what has gotten you upset. Many times, all you need to do is to make a change in the way you are doing or thinking about something.

Focusing on your breath and breathing diaphragmatically can also get you through uncomfortable or difficult procedures such as magnetic resonance imaging (MRI), pelvic exams, sigmoidoscopies, and injections. In fact, many of life's challenges can be made a little easier by just breathing. Make breath-focusing exercises a part of your daily routine.

Mini-Relaxations

When you take a moment and focus on diaphragmatic breathing, think of this as a "mini-relaxation." Begin to practice mini-relaxations during the day to release tension that has accumulated over short periods of time. Here are some suggestions for different kinds of mini-relaxations:

1. Whenever you have just a minute, take a deep breath; as you breathe out, imagine all the tension in your body and mind leaving through this breath.

2. Take a moment to tense all the muscles you can at once. Then take a deep breath and slowly breathe out, letting all the tension go. Take another deep breath and reduce the tension further. Repeat until the tension is gone.

3. Take an inventory of body tension in your familiar stress points. For example, is there tension in your neck or upper back? If you find that there is, pretend that you can direct the breath into that area of tension. As you breathe out, feel the tension release.

4. Count to 10 taking a slow, deep breath. Hold the breath for one count. Then breathe out slowly, again as you count to 10.

Preparing to Practice Eliciting the RR

Minimizing Distractions and Making Yourself Comfortable

Plan to practice an RR technique for 20 minutes once a day, or for 10 minutes twice a day. Pick a time to do your RR practice when your pain is not at its worst. To minimize distractions, find a quiet, comfortable place where you feel safe practicing the RR techniques described later.

If necessary, put a "Do Not Disturb" sign (provided at the end of this book) on the door and take the phone off the hook.

By all means, respect your need for comfort and find the position that feels best to you. The following are suggestions for making yourself comfortable:

- Use a heating pad, ice, and/or supportive pillows to make yourself as comfortable as needed.

- Make sure the temperature in the room is right for you, or have a blanket nearby if you should become chilled.

- If you prefer to lie down while eliciting the RR but find yourself falling asleep, try a sitting position. A good compromise between lying down and sitting is using a reclining chair.

- When you end your session, always count to three and slowly open your eyes. Get up slowly, so that your body will adjust to the postural change after such deep relaxation.

- Do not set an alarm. If you are not using a relaxation tape and want to keep track of the time, just set a clock in front of you and open your eyes periodically. After practicing a few times, you will usually be able to judge when 20 minutes have elapsed.

Using Relaxation Tapes

Relaxation or meditation CDs, tapes, or MP3 downloads can be quite valuable when you are first learning an RR technique. Tapes of environmental sounds and music for meditation are also available through local or online bookstores, and some people find it helpful to make their own relaxation tape to guide them.

I have recorded three guided relaxation exercises for pain that you can use with this book. They are available for free download from the publisher's website (*www.guilford.com/managepain*). Have this book handy when you go to download; the website will ask you to type in a password from the book. Just follow the directions. These audio exercises correspond to RR techniques described a bit later in this chapter. Look for the headphones graphic next to those techniques with audios.

What you use to help stay focused is not as important as staying as focused as you can in a relaxed and nonjudgmental way. My colleagues and I recommend that in the beginning you keep to a simple technique (see "Basic RR Techniques," later in this chapter). Changing tracks, tapes, or focus word(s) every other day will not help you focus your mind. Consistency is important when you are first learning a technique. Use a tape (or word, phrase, or breath) for some time before deciding that you need to make a change.

Mind Chatter

At times your thoughts may feel as if they are going off in many different directions. The resulting chatter of your mind may go on and on, sounding like a cast of thousands. This can be very distracting and it can affect your concentration. This is normal; it happens to all of us; it shows us that we can sometimes be one place mentally and another place physically. You may be thinking about something that happened in the past or planning for the future. It's difficult not to get caught up in these random thoughts.

There is a time and place for this "mind chatter," but it always seems to get louder when you are trying to practice an RR technique. Mind chatter is persistent, and you may find that it creeps into your consciousness even as you assume a passive attitude. Just keep gently returning your attention to your breath or your focus word (see RR Technique 1, in the next section). With practice, focus on the repeated breath or word can reduce mind chatter or even temporarily eliminate it.

Problem Solving

You may encounter obstacles that keep you from practicing the RR techniques. No doubt you can always find a hundred reasons not to do your RR practice. This section could be called "No Excuses!"

The following are the most common problems that participants have in this program. After reading this section, you should feel better able to handle any obstacles that prevent you from practicing the RR techniques.

Lack of Time

"I don't have the time!" you may exclaim. The response is simple: If you want to feel better, *make* the time. First, ask yourself why you feel you don't have the time. Do these answers from previous program participants seem familiar?

> "What will people think if they see me doing nothing? I do so little as it is."
>
> "My family needs me."
>
> "This can't possibly make a difference—my pain is real."
>
> "I'm in too much pain."

Statements like these may come from giving too much control to others, from low self-esteem or learned helplessness, or simply from practicing at times when your pain is at its worst or you're too exhausted. These are all normal feelings, but you won't feel any better if you let them stop you. Your choice is "to do or not to do." When you choose "to do," you have the opportunity to experience all the positive benefits of bringing about the RR and reducing your stress.

Increased Awareness of Pain

You may find, as have many other people, that you are more aware of your pain when you minimize distractions and try to practice an RR technique. Sometimes when you close your eyes in a quiet room, the pain comes roaring back.

Try finding a comfortable position that reduces your pain as much as possible. If this fails, practice RR Technique 6 (self-hypnosis), described later in this chapter. Sometimes just focusing all of your attention on the pain will at first increase it, but within seconds this awareness should diminish. The brain is not "wired" to pay attention to things that do not change.

In his book *Full Catastrophe Living* (see "Supplementary Reading" at the end of this chapter), Jon Kabat-Zinn describes a meditation technique called "mindfulness." This technique encourages you to let the mind stay passively focused on the pain. Allow yourself simply to observe the pain and the feelings you may have, such as fear or anger, without running away from those feelings or the sensation. Say to yourself, "Oh, yes, that's my pain and that's my anger." This technique can have dramatic results. When you stay passively focused on the pain you begin to realize how much you fight your pain and avoid your feelings about it, both of which increase your feelings of powerlessness. Once you understand this, then every time the pain tugs at your awareness during the practice, you may find you do not have to fight it. You do not have feed it with anger, anxiety, or frustration. You can simply return to your focus word, phrase, or breath. This technique may seem impossible. You may want to ignore your pain because you may fear it will get worse. It will not. This technique is a very powerful way to grasp the fact that the pain exists and that you are the one who experiences the pain. How you choose to feel about your pain is under your control.

Problems with Sitting Still or Relaxing

You may say, "I can't sit still. I'm not the kind of person to relax; I must be busy. I feel anxious when I start to relax or close my eyes." If this is so, ask yourself why you can't sit still.

To begin with, do you like your own company? Do you feel worthwhile only if you're doing something? Some people have such a fragile sense of self-worth and self-esteem that they are the last people they want to sit with. In fact, they don't like their own company. Some people feel that meeting others' demands is the only activity that counts. This makes sitting quietly and bringing about the RR seem like an "irresponsible" thing to do. Still others may be so physically tense that they don't know what it's like to relax (in mind or body!).

If you are physically tense, try some gentle stretching. Systematic contracting and relaxing of various muscle groups, as in "progressive muscle relaxation" (see RR Technique 3 in the next section), may also be helpful. If your self-esteem is low or your need to meet others' demands is high, you may find the following recommendation helpful. At the beginning of your RR practice, take a moment to imagine a covered basket or toolbox sitting beside you. Identify the thoughts that are going through your head that are causing worry or concern. As you identify these items, imagine opening the basket or toolbox and depositing the items. Make an agreement with yourself that you can take all those things out right after you do your RR session, but while you are in the RR practice, they are to remain where you've put them. It is surprising how effective this simple negotiation with yourself can be. *You* can decide when you will or won't be distracted or worried.

Some people have trouble relaxing because they are trying to avoid memories of traumatic events, such as physical or sexual abuse. This inability to relax is associated with hypervigilance (being on guard against harm) and has been described in various posttraumatic stress syndromes. For some, these traumatic memories surface whenever they let their guard down and relax. For others, these memories have been hidden from consciousness until they started to practice the RR techniques.

My colleagues and I have found that these memories needn't keep someone from enjoying the benefits of the RR. There are ways of modifying the RR techniques to minimize the anxiety (see below). Furthermore, because reactions to past trauma tend to magnify negative feelings about chronic pain—of vulnerability, of being out of control, of feeling that "no one believes me"—it is important to separate the experiences of previous trauma and present chronic pain.

It is not possible to give universal recommendations for the very complicated reactions people can have to trauma. However, the following suggestions might help decrease the discomfort of these feelings.

1. Acknowledge that you are indeed a very special person for having taken the initiative to pick up this book. Parts of you sense that things have not been going well and that there must be a better way. Hang on to this self-awareness; it can get you through the rough times. Change is not easy and rarely proceeds without effort.

2. Practice your RR techniques in a safe place, with locked doors and the lights on if necessary. Do whatever it takes to make yourself feel comfortable. Sometimes if you create a safe physical environment, you can begin to feel safe inside.

3. Use a relaxation tape to minimize internal distractions. Keep your eyes open or stare at a candle flame as a focus. Do progressive muscle relaxation or use an exercise that couples movement and breath focus. This, too, will help cut down on the internal distractions.

4. Biofeedback therapy can sometimes be very helpful. While you are learning to relax it gives you external feedback on your internal processes—such as muscle tension, skin conductance, and skin temperature. Biofeedback devices keep your attention focused on changing these physical parameters until you are comfortable enough to do so on your own without the machine.

5. Psychotherapy with someone experienced at treating posttraumatic stress syndromes can also support your efforts. In my experience, once trauma memories surface, they will not be pushed out of consciousness again. However, their conscious presence may mean that you are now ready to deal with the memories. If possible, try to come to terms with your past experiences and memories. They do have an impact on your pain and can cause serious stress in their own right. *Seek help and take care of yourself.*

Peculiar Sensations or Experiences

Although it is a rare complaint, some program participants have reported out-of-body experiences, dissociation, or feelings of a presence other than their own. In most of these cases, the persons have been practicing an RR technique for longer than recommended—more than 1 hour, or several times a day for an hour or more. This is an instance in which doing something more, or more often, is not necessarily better for you. Overuse of such techniques can lead to alterations in consciousness, and it is therefore important to follow the specific instructions provided. The techniques presented in the next section are safe and very effective if used as instructed.

Some people are so used to feeling "wired" that feeling relaxed feels peculiar to them. If this is the case for you, you may just need to learn what it feels like to be relaxed.

Seizure Disorders

If you have a seizure disorder, it is suggested that you practice your RR techniques while lying down. Some seizures are brought on by a change in level of arousal, such as going to sleep or awakening. Because the brain waves associated with bringing about the RR are similar to those occurring in the first stage of sleep, people with rare sleep-onset seizure disorders may experience their seizures when they first start practicing. This may pass with continued practice or with the use of another technique (progressive muscle relaxation, yoga, or another physically focused repetitive technique). Some people have found that they can actually help *control* their seizures by practicing the RR techniques, learning to relax, and redirecting their focus of attention with the first sign of a coming seizure. *If you have questions, check with your doctor.*

Insulin-Dependent Diabetes

Adrenaline can alter insulin availability, making it necessary for more insulin to be in circulation. Therefore, stress can increase the amount of insulin you need. Many patients on insulin find that they need less insulin after starting regular practice of an RR technique. If you are an insulin-dependent diabetic, take hypoglycemic reactions *seriously* and reduce your insulin intake if you begin to experience lower blood sugar levels. *Check with your doctor.*

Hypertension

Blood pressure medications can interfere with the body's normal adjustments to changes in posture. If you take drugs for hypertension, make sure you change positions *slowly* when getting up after your RR practice, whether from lying to sitting or from sitting to standing. Many patients find that with regular practice of RR techniques, their blood pressure may decrease, and their medication requirements may even be reduced. *Be sure to check with your physician before making any ad-justments in your medication(s).*

Basic RR Techniques

Now that you know what RR is, how to prepare for it, and what to expect, you can start learning some basic techniques for bringing it about. It is important that you start with the basic techniques and master those before moving on to the more advanced ones.

To practice the following techniques, begin by finding yourself a quiet, comfortable position in which your body can relax.

Close your eyes (unless that is uncomfortable or unsafe—as it would be if you were walking, as in Technique 4) and begin to focus as directed on a word or phrase, on your breath, or on creating muscle tension. When you are distracted by your thoughts or pain gently guide your mind back to the focus.

RR Technique 1: Using a Focus Word or Phrase

Focus your mind on repeating a word or short phrase with each out-breath. What word or phrase you choose is less important than its repetition. Remember that this is just a way of keeping your mind focused. You can use the number "one," or count to 10 repetitively with each breath, or count "one" on the in-breath and "two" on the out-breath.

You can also just find a sound that is comforting to say. If you have a religious or spiritual preference or practice, a short prayer or phrase can be used. I do recommend, however, that you avoid words or phrases like "Go! Go! Go!" or "I must relax!" With such phrases, you are pressuring yourself to do more and more in less and less time. This is not the intention of RR techniques. The aim is not for you to do more of what you have been doing in the way you've been doing it, but to take the time to sit and focus. This allows your natural body wisdom to be restored.

If you find your mind wandering, gently guide it back to your focus word or phrase.

RR Technique 2: Coupling Breathing with Imagination

Use your breath coupled with your imagination. This exercise is sometimes helpful to those who find focusing on their chests or abdomens too uncomfortable or anxiety-provoking.

For example, you can picture your breath coming in through your right hand and out through your left hand, or in and out through your right hand. "Breathing" through your feet can also be used. Or you can imagine the in-breath going to areas of tension such as your face, neck, or back; as you breathe out, imagine the breath and tension disappearing into the air. Each time a breath goes out, feel yourself becoming more relaxed.

Ocean Sounds. Another version of this technique can be found on the Ocean Sounds relaxation audio available for free download at the publisher's website (*www.guilford.com/managepain*). This 20-minute recording starts with a focus on the body to orient your attention and then guides your imagination to images of a beach; ocean sounds then play. You may find that your breath naturally flows with the rhythm of the ocean waves, in and out, like the waves on the beach. If you practice with this track once a day, you will get the recommended 20 minutes of daily RR practice.

RR Technique 3: Progressive Muscle Relaxation

Alternately tensing and relaxing various parts of the body is another helpful technique for individuals who find it difficult to relax by sitting quietly.

You can reduce distraction by engaging in physical and mental focusing. For example, curl the toes of your right foot on the in-breath, and relax them on the out-breath. Next, flex your right foot back toward your head on the in-breath, and then relax the foot on the out-breath. Then straighten your right leg at the knee on the in-breath and relax the knee on the out-breath. Tense your right buttock on the in-breath and relax it on the out-breath. Repeat the sequence for the left leg, and progress up the body until all parts have been tensed and relaxed in sequence with the breath.

There are progressive relaxation tapes available that can guide you in this technique. (See "Using Relaxation Tapes" in the previous section.)

RR Technique 4: Using Repetitive Motion

Perform a repetitive motion while coupling your breath and mind with the motion. For instance, running, swimming, stationary bicycling, or using a treadmill can be used to elicit the RR, as long as your breath and mind are in sync with the movement.

As an example, let's suppose that you are walking on a treadmill. You can inhale on two steps and exhale on two steps repetitively and focus on that breath–movement rhythm. Of course, the ratio of breath to steps will depend on your level of conditioning, comfort, and speed. When you find yourself distracted from the rhythm of your breath and movement by thoughts, gently return your focus to your breath and movement.

Yoga and tai chi are also effective ways of coupling breath, mind, and motion. Such techniques involving ritualized posturing of the body were used to bring about the RR in ancient cultures.

RR Technique 5: Creating a Safe Place

Many people in pain feel betrayed by their bodies. Pain can make you feel trapped with nowhere to hide or find comfort. It is possible, by using your various senses, to re-create a safe haven in your mind. Some program participants have reported strong, pleasant, and familiar odors while they are in their safe places; others have tactile (touch) sensations of warmth and softness. Everyone has different experiences. You should allow your favorite and most comforting sensations to be present—sound, smell, touch, sight, or a combination of the senses. A guided imagery audio version of this technique can be downloaded for free from *www.guilford.com/managepain*.

The following exercise has been one of the most beneficial versions of this fifth basic RR technique for people in pain:

1. Begin by engaging in one of the first three basic RR techniques.

2. When you are focused and relaxed, create an image in your mind that feels safe and comforting. Your safe place can be somewhere you went as a child, a pleasant vacation spot, or a place you saw in a book. It can be a favorite room in your home, your bed, or an imagined large fluffy cloud. You can move the mountains next to the seashore or create a totally bug-free forest scene . . . wherever your imagination leads. The key here is to envision a place associated with peace and comfort.

3. When you have imagined your special place, find a comfortable spot to sit or lie and pass some quality time here, repeating your focus word or phrase with each breath. When you become distracted by thoughts, gently guide your awareness back to your focus.

4. Enjoy the experience!

With practice, you can re-create this image by focusing on your breath or the words "safe place" whenever you need some respite.

Advanced RR Techniques

The advanced RR techniques described here allow you to obtain additional results and insights. However, if you are inexperienced in achieving the RR, you may feel uncomfortable at the images that come into your head during the visualization exercise (Technique 7). You should have first practiced and become skilled at creating a safe place inside yourself. For many people in chronic pain, the pain is a beast or a big dark cloud, which can be quite intimidating (and scary) if not approached from a position of experience with the basic techniques. Or you may feel anxious about the instructions to create numbness and an absence of feeling in certain body areas during the self-hypnosis exercise (Technique 6). Therefore, it is recommended that you practice the advanced techniques *only* after you have had experience eliciting the RR by means of the basic techniques, especially Technique 5 (creating a safe place).

RR Technique 6: Self-Hypnosis

The following is a simple self-hypnosis exercise. Begin by performing one of the basic RR techniques that you have learned. Once you are feeling relaxed, proceed as follows:

1. Close your eyes and imagine that your right hand is becoming pleasantly warm and heavy. Each time you breathe out, the pleasant sensation of warmth and heaviness becomes greater, until your hand feels so heavy it can hardly move (unless you want it to).

2. Now feel a pleasant numbness that begins in your right thumb, then moves to your second finger, the third finger, the fourth finger, and finally the fifth finger with each out-breath. The numbness spreads to the palm of your right hand and then to the back of the hand, stopping at the wrist. It is a pleasant, warm, heavy, and numb sensation only in your right hand.

3. Either physically place your right hand on your painful area, or imagine that the numbness in your right hand is moving there. When all the numbness has been absorbed into the area of pain, return to your focus word or breath. When you are ready to end this session, transfer the numbness back to your right hand.

4. Now feel the normal sensations coming into the back of your right hand, then the palm, the fifth finger, the fourth finger, the third finger, the second finger, and the thumb. Your hand still feels warm and heavy.

5. Gradually feel your hand becoming lighter and lighter with each breath. Feel it become normal, just like your left hand.

6. Count to three and open your eyes.

The more you practice this technique, the more quickly you can develop the sensation of numbness, which can be transferred to the area of pain. You can also make your own tape with these instructions to help you master this technique.

This is a technique that can temporarily alter the pain experience. If you wish to explore hypnosis further, there are psychotherapists who have special training and certification in hypnosis who may help you identify other techniques that might suit your needs better. An inspiring story about how one person used hypnosis to control his pain can be found in *A Whole New Life* by Reynolds Price (see "Supplementary Reading" at the end of this chapter).

RR Technique 7: Pain Control Visualization

In this visualization exercise you create and work with an image of your pain. You may find my audio recording of this technique helpful. It can be downloaded from the publisher's website (*www.guilford.com/managepain*).

As noted earlier, this technique should not be attempted without experience with the basic RR techniques, especially Technique 5, because many people's images of their pain can be quite frightening. If your image gets too scary, just open your eyes; remember that you have control over it.

> Gail suffered from terrible migraines that were occurring at least once a week. During the visualization exercise she saw her pain as a red, hot ball that pulsated. When asked to modify the pain in some way, she decided to build an igloo around it, and the red ball turned blue.
>
> The next time Gail started to get her usual warning of the headache to come, she closed her eyes, imagined the red, hot ball, and then built an igloo around it until it turned blue. The headache didn't come! Gail was able to stop many of her headaches with this technique.

To begin this exercise, again, engage in one of the basic RR techniques. When you feel focused and relaxed, create an image in your mind in the following manner:

1. Imagine yourself in a meadow where the sun is shining, it's not too hot or too cool, and a gentle breeze is blowing.

2. Picture a path. As you walk along it, a sense of safety and security accompanies you. In the distance you can hear the birds singing in the trees, and you can smell the sweet scent of wildflowers. Follow the path across a bridge to a house that sits at the edge of the meadow.

3. Walk up the steps of the house and open the front door. When you walk inside, you will find a large room divided into two parts by a large wall made of clear, impenetrable plastic. This wall extends from floor to ceiling and from one end of the room to the other.

4. Make yourself comfortable and sit in front of the clear plastic wall.

5. Gather up your pain into a ball. Take this ball of pain and notice that the clear plastic wall in front of you opens up to let you drop the pain on the other side. After you have placed the pain on the other side, the wall closes up again, and the pain must remain there until you instruct it otherwise.

6. Give your pain a color, a shape, or a form. It can be a symbol of what your pain feels like, or it can be like a cartoon character.

7. Now observe its behavior. Does it bounce around, scream, or look menacing? How does being face to face with it make you feel?

8. Ask your pain these questions and listen to the responses:

    "Why are you here?"

    "What can I learn from you?"

    "When will you go away?"

    "Can we coexist together?"

9. You can ask the pain any other questions that you may have. Most people have a lot of questions to ask or things to say to their pain when given this opportunity.

10. Now think about how you might change the image of your pain in some way. For example, if it looks like a blob that is ill defined, pour it into a container and give it boundaries. You don't have to destroy it; just let your ideas and the image come freely. If it's hot, cool it down. If it's sharp, dull the edges. As you try different approaches, ask yourself how you feel about manipulating your pain. Is there any effect on your pain as you try these different approaches?

11. When you are finished asking questions and/or modifying your pain, make one of the following decisions:

    Take all of the pain back.

    Leave all of the pain behind the clear plastic wall.

    Take part of the pain back.

12. Once you have made your decision, walk out the front door of the house and close it behind you.

13. Walk down the front steps and into the sunshine. Move along the path, over the bridge, and back into the meadow again.

14. Take the path to your safe place where you have established a haven of refuge and solace (Technique 5). Spend some time there focusing your mind and releasing any residual tension.

15. When you are finished, open your eyes.

This technique can be a very powerful emotional experience. It can be used to examine any problem, not just your pain. By removing or distancing yourself from the pain or other problem, you can get a fresh outlook, and new solutions can be explored.

Dorothy was amazed. The image before her was as gray and ominous as anything she had ever felt in all the years she had pain. It had no edges or boundaries. The pain looked like smoky wisps that crept along the edges of the clear wall, as if it were trying to find an opening to escape.

Dorothy asked it questions but received no answers. Her pain remained as elusive as it had always been. What wasn't elusive, however, was the sense of impending doom she felt whenever the pain increased.

Dorothy continued to practice this technique and always created a safe place after confronting her pain. As she began exploring the pain with her pain diary and some of the cognitive exercises (see Chapter 5), she started to see images that were more concrete and defined. At first she saw a ghost, then a character that

> looked like the Michelin tire man. One day she was able to pump the tire man up until it exploded into a thousand pieces.
>
> Dorothy then felt a sense of release and relief. She realized that the fear of the pain had held her a prisoner; once she became able to face this fear, she was able to feel less controlled by it.

The use of imagery allows you to explore the nonverbal, unconscious experience of pain meanings and metaphors. It can help you make connections to other experiences or perceptions that might not be reached through logical reasoning. This, in turn, can give you an entirely different attitude toward your pain. It can expand your control of the pain experience.

Another way of looking at the effects of this exercise is to place your hand over your face with fingers spread apart. Your vision is impaired, and you are not able to see the back of your hand. Now, as your hand moves away from your face, you can see more details, and there is more freedom to turn your hand around to see both the back and the front. Similarly, distancing pain or other problems behind the plastic wall allows you to see a greater range of solutions for the problems that may confront you.

Summary

Chronic Pain as Chronic Stress; The RR

- Chronic pain fits the definition of chronic stress. Chronic stress makes it difficult for you to reestablish homeostasis (balance). It can exhaust your body's ability to restore itself to normal.
- Practicing techniques that bring about the relaxation response (RR) will help your body recover from chronic stress.
- The RR is a natural bodily response, but it requires training and practice. It involves (1) focusing your mind on a repeated phrase, word, breath, or action; and (2) adopting a passive attitude toward interfering thoughts.

Breathing and Breathing Exercises

- The key to bringing about the RR is focused awareness; you can focus on your breathing.
- There are two types of breathing:
    - —Chest breathing: with each in-breath, your chest expands.
    - —Diaphragmatic breathing: with each in-breath, your abdomen expands.
- Become aware of how you breathe.

- If you are a chest breather, relearn diaphragmatic breathing with the three exercises in this chapter.

- Once you're aware of your breathing, start to practice breath focusing. It encourages you to focus on the present, the here and now. Focus on your breathing can release tension, decrease pain, and increase control.

- Take a moment during the day to focus on breathing; think of it a "mini-relaxation."

Preparing to Practice Eliciting the RR

- Minimize distractions and make yourself as comfortable as possible while you practice the RR techniques.

- Relaxation tapes can be quite helpful in learning to bring about the RR. If you plan to use relaxation tapes, don't continually change them; be consistent with your object of focus, particularly when you first begin.

- "Mind chatter" is the name for all the thoughts going through your mind. This chatter is perfectly normal but it can distract you from your focus. Just keep gently returning your focus to your repeated breath, word, phrase, or action. With practice, you can reduce the chatter and perhaps even eliminate it temporarily.

- In the beginning, many obstacles may keep you from practicing the RR techniques; however, these techniques are critical to overcoming your pain and succeeding with this program. So, in the interest of better health, remember the following:

  —If you want to feel better, make the time to practice the techniques.

  —Your pain may get worse during practice, but you can develop your ability to focus and decrease the pain.

  —If you have trouble with sitting still or relaxing because of physical tension, try gentle stretching or progressive muscle relaxation; if you have low self-esteem or a strong need to meet others' demands, try imagining that you put your worries in a basket while you practice.

  —If you are dealing with posttraumatic stress (for example, sexual abuse memories), you can modify the techniques in various ways to minimize your anxiety and decrease your discomfort. Seek additional professional help if you are feeling overwhelmed.

  —If you have peculiar sensations or experiences (for example, out-of-body experiences, dissociation) while practicing an RR technique, you may be practicing too long or too often.

  —If you have a seizure disorder, diabetes, or hypertension, you need to know how RR techniques may affect you. Be sure to read the relevant section of this chapter and learn what you may need to do to accommodate your disorder.

Basic RR Techniques

- Technique 1: Mentally focus on repeating a word or short phrase on each out-breath.
- Technique 2: Use your breath, coupled with your imagination. Picture your in-breath going into the areas of tension, and on the out-breath, let the tension go.
- Technique 3: Alternately tense and relax various parts of your body (this is called progressive muscle relaxation).
- Technique 4: Keep repeating a motion in sync with the rhythm of your breath as your mind focuses on it.
- Technique 5: Create a safe haven in your mind where you can leave your pain behind and go to rest.

Advanced RR Techniques

- Practice these two advanced RR techniques only after you have become skilled in the basic RR techniques (1–5).
  - —Technique 6: This simple self-hypnosis technique allows you to transfer sensations from one part of your body to another.
  - —Technique 7: This visualization technique allows you to place your pain behind a clear wall; give it a form; ask it questions; modify its form and study the effect on your pain; and then decide whether to take part, all, or none of it back. Not only can this technique be a very powerful emotional experience, it can also be extremely effective, and you can put any problem behind the clear plastic wall.

Exploration Tasks

1. Practice your goal-setting skills by writing out a goal that involves one of the RR techniques. Make sure that your goal meets the criteria set forth in Chapter 1—in other words, that it is a realistic behavioral task that can be measured in the steps that *you* will take to accomplish it. Here is an example:

   Goal: <u>*Practice RR Technique 1 once a day.*</u>

   Steps to take to reach that goal:

   A. <u>*Take phone off hook.*</u>

   B. <u>*Use the recliner to maximize comfort.*</u>

   C. <u>*Practice as soon as I get out of bed.*</u>

In addition, list contingency plans. Making contingency plans is a way of troubleshooting before a problem occurs. Thinking ahead of time about what might get in the way of achieving your goal can help you develop strategies to solve the problem. Here is an example:

Obstacles	**Solutions**
A. <u>*Can't relax, pain too bad*</u>	<u>*Listen to RR tape, practice in bathtub*</u>
B. <u>*Family members disturb me*</u>	<u>*Hang "Do Not Disturb" sign on door*</u>

Now it's your turn.

Goal: _____

Steps to take to reach that goal:

A. _____

B. _____

C. _____

D. _____

List contingency plans. What steps can you take to work toward insuring your success?

Obstacles	**Solutions**
A. _____	_____
B. _____	_____
C. _____	_____
D. _____	_____

2. Practice diaphragmatic breathing as frequently as possible, both during the day and before going to sleep.

3. In the midst of tension, increased pain, or emotional distress, remember to do the following:

A. Consciously stop and pause.

B. Take a deep, slow breath from your diaphragm.

C. Reflect on the situation and your choices.

4. Incorporate "mini-relaxations" into your daily routine.

When do you do mini-relaxations? _____

What techniques do you use? _____

_____

What can you do to remind yourself to do mini-relaxations throughout the day? _____

_____

5. Practice an RR technique once a day for 20 minutes. In the beginning, don't be concerned with breathing diaphragmatically; just breathe your normal way. Practice the diaphragmatic breathing separately. Practice one of the basic techniques (1–5) daily for at least 5 weeks before moving on to the advanced techniques (6–7). Again, it is important to be comfortable with the basic techniques before using the more advanced techniques.

6. Complete the RR technique diary at the back of the book. Next to each category, indicate the appropriate information about your daily practice. Use this diary for the first 3 weeks to reinforce practice.

Supplementary Reading

The following books provide additional information on the mind–body connection in general and the RR in particular:

Herbert Benson, *The Relaxation Response* (New York: HarperCollins, 2000).
Joan Borysenko, *Minding the Body, Mending the Mind* (New York: Da Capo Press, 2007).
Patrick Fanning, *Visualization for Change* (Oakland, CA: New Harbinger Publications, 1994).
Shakti Gawain, *Creative Visualization* (New York: New World Library, 2002).
Thich Nhat Hanh, *The Miracle of Mindfulness: A Manual of Meditation* (Boston: Beacon Press, 1996).
Jon Kabat-Zinn, *Arriving at Your Own Door: 108 Lessons in Mindfulness* (New York: Hyperion, 2007).
Jon Kabat-Zinn, *Full Catastrophe Living: Using the Wisdom of Your Body and Mind to Face Stress, Pain, and Illness* (New York: Delacorte Press, 1990).
Reynolds Price, *A Whole New Life* (New York: Scribner, 2000).
Madisyn Taylor, *Daily OM: Inspirational Thoughts for a Happy, Healthy and Fulfilling Day* (Carlsbad, CA: Hay House, 2008).

4

The Body–Mind Connection

Chapter 3 explored how your mind can affect your body. Now let's take a look at how your body can affect your mind.

When you are in pain, you may tend to do the following:

- Ignore all sensation from the neck down or label all sensation as painful.
- Stop moving your body parts except when it's absolutely necessary.
- Withdraw from social interactions.
- Push yourself physically by denying your condition.

These attitudes and behaviors need to be challenged. They either feed your fear of activity or make you do far too much. When you stop moving, you lose muscle strength and endurance; when you do too much you can reinjure yourself. You can become isolated, lonely, and depressed. One patient, John, has described all of this well in the following story.

> I used to get up in the morning with the challenge of doing things as usual, in spite of my pain. Maybe today would be different. Sure, the pain was my issue, but I was also getting subtle and not-so-subtle messages from my family and friends: "It used to be so much fun when you could do this. . . . Remember when you could do that? . . . When are you going back to work? It might get your mind off your problems."
>
> I felt it was impossible to explain. No one understood. Even I had a difficult time understanding why my back continued to spasm with the least amount of activity. I was terrified of doing things for fear of making the pain worse; yet, at the same time, I was ashamed because I couldn't even keep up with the laundry. How could I ever drive a truck again—the only thing I knew how to do for a living? So each day I would push myself through the odd jobs at home and collapse at the end of the day, with the pain worse than ever.
>
> So what did I accomplish? I became more irritable, depressed, and with-

drawn. I felt trapped and alone. My children tiptoed past me as I lay on the couch, and my wife and I constantly bickered. One day I found her sobbing. She told me that she felt she had lost her best friend and husband to the pain. I made the decision there and then to seek help, and found this program.

Your body can become a resource for you, instead of something to ignore or push into submission. When you learn to listen to your body, it can tell you how to pace yourself, how to plan your activities, so that you do more with less pain. Becoming aware of when you are in pain allows you to use your body to change your mood and sensations. You can begin to do more things that give you pleasure; you can have a life again. This chapter will show you how to do all these things.

Increasing Activities

Pain can prevent you from moving comfortably. It can make working and having fun more difficult, if not downright impossible. Through keeping your diary, you may be starting to see how your pain is influenced by what you do and how what you do is influenced by your pain. Keeping active while in pain requires you to use three strategies:

- Pacing
- Adaptation
- Delegation

Pacing is about conserving your energy over the long haul. It means not letting the stress of pain and overactivity exhaust you. Instead of "sprinting" through an activity, you "walk." Instead of working harder, you work smarter. Using this approach, you are more likely to get a task done without increasing your pain and suffering. Pacing activities can reduce fatigue and spasm (which increase pain) because the body isn't pushed to exhaustion. Pushing yourself to the point of exhaustion can increase tension, inflammation, and nerve irritation.

Pacing is based on observing what positions (such as sitting or standing) or activities (such as vacuuming or combing your hair) increase your pain after what period of time. For example, do you know how long you can stand before your pain goes from a 4 to a 6 on the pain scale from Chapter 1? Knowing when your pain is getting worse gives you an idea of how long you can stand to do the dishes before you sit and pay your bills. How long do you have to sit before the pain goes back down to 4, where it was before the dishes? Pacing is about knowing your limits, so you can then alternate sitting with standing activities, get more accomplished, and not increase your pain and exhaustion. It's good to use a timer or other reminder. Even so, you have to control the temptation to do one more dish. Let's take a look at John's usual day before starting this program and his usual day now, as an example.

Then		Now	
9 A.M.	Get up **Pain sensation = 6** **Emotional response = 7**	7 A.M.	Get up **Pain sensation = 5** **Emotional response = 3**
9:30 A.M.	Breakfast	7:30 A.M.	Stretching, relaxation technique
10:30 A.M.	Do the dishes, watch TV	8:30 A.M.	Shower, get dressed
11 A.M.	Lie down	9 A.M.	Get bills together to pay
1 P.M.	Get up and eat lunch	9:15 A.M.	Wash dishes for 10 minutes
1:30 P.M.	Work on the car (Pain = 7)	9:25 A.M.	Pay bills for 15 minutes
3:00 P.M.	Pick up children	9:40 A.M.	Bring laundry down in four small bundles
4:30 P.M.	Eat dinner		
5:00 P.M.	Watch TV	10 A.M.	Log on Internet for support group
7:00 P.M.	Go to bed **Pain sensation = 8** **Emotional response = 7**	10:20 A.M.	Start wash in washing machine
		11 A.M.	Finish bills
		11:30 A.M.	Finish dishes
		Noon	Eat lunch
		12:30 P.M.	Put wet clothes in dryer
		1:00 P.M.	Peel vegetables for dinner
		1:45 P.M.	Take dry clothes out of dryer
		2:15 P.M.	Fold clothes while sitting
		3 P.M.	Pick up children at school
		3:15–6 P.M.	Watch soccer game
		6:15 P.M.	Set table
		6:30 P.M.	Eat dinner
		7:00 P.M.	Stretches
		7:30 P.M.	Help children with homework
		9:00 P.M.	Read bedtime story
		9:30 P.M.	Hot shower and bed **Pain sensation = 5** **Emotional response = 3**

Adaptation means finding new (less painful) ways to accomplish old tasks. For example, there is no rule that dishes have to be done in the sink or clothes folded while standing. It's quite all right to sit to do dishes in a dishpan or to fold clothes. Put a bench in the shower or bathtub so you can sit and scrub. Use shoes with Velcro clasps. Put large-handle grips on stirring spoons and pens. These are all ways to make your life more comfortable. Such gadgets and ideas can be obtained from your local hospital's occupational therapy department. Share ideas with members of your local pain support group or on the Internet.

Delegation is another way to conserve your energy. It's like job sharing. "If you carry the laundry upstairs, I'll fold it." "If you get the bills together, I'll pay them." "You clean the bathrooms; I'll pick up the living room." Entertain by hosting potlucks—everyone brings a dish. Tell guests that if they volunteer to wash or dry dishes, they don't have to prepare anything! Can't do a certain task? Ask a friend. They may have something you can do for them in return—and don't forget to pace yourself!

Pacing, adaptation, and delegation allow you the most flexibility while acknowledging that your pain is real but that techniques for managing it can be incorporated into your life.

Dealing with Difficulties in Changing the Way You Do Your Activities

You may, of course, be able to think of any number of reasons for not pacing yourself or altering your routines:

"I don't do enough as it is. How can I take a break?"

"I have to do things like everyone else, or at least like my mother [or father] did."

"I'm too busy to take a break. What will my family do?"

"I can't ask for help, understanding, or a change in schedule."

"My pain is always the same no matter what I do."

It may be difficult for you to take the lead in deciding what you can and cannot do (instead of living up to others' expectations). As this book states repeatedly, however, it is absolutely essential that *you* take control. No one else can judge what you are able or not able to do.

The following story shows why it's so important to examine what you do and why you do it.

A woman was busy fixing a Sunday pot roast. She cut off the ends of the roast in her preparation. He daughter watched as she did this and asked why she cut the ends off.

"Well," she said after some contemplation, "that's how my mother used to prepare it. Let's call Grammy and ask her."

She called her mother and asked.

Her mother replied, "Hmmm. . . . I guess I never thought about it before because my mother, your grandmother, always did it."

Curious now as to what the answer might be, the woman called her grandmother to solve this culinary mystery. In response to the question, her grand-

---

> mother laughed and laughed. "I used to cut off the ends of the pot roast because it was always too big to fit into the tiny roasting pan that fit in my little oven of 50 years ago!"

By examining what you do, you can decide what you want to keep and what you want to discard—like the ends of a pot roast. Once you have determined what *you need* (as opposed to what others expect), I recommend that you tell those around you. Other people will generally be supportive of changes in your routines if you explain why you want to make them. They certainly will welcome your being in a better mood because you're in less discomfort.

> Martha decided that she could stand to do dishes at the sink for only 5 minutes before she needed to sit down. She arranged to use her oven timer to cue her when the 5 minutes were up. She also arranged to have some stationery and her address book on the kitchen table, so that she could catch up on correspondence; she would do this for 10 minutes while she sat and "rested." At first the other members of her family did not understand. Some wondered why she was "goofing off" in this way; others kept trying to finish the dishes for her when they saw her sit down. Martha was able to tell them that this was what she needed to do for herself and reminded them (and herself) that there was no rule limiting dishwashing to any specific period of time. She felt better about accomplishing this task by herself, and because of her pacing she experienced no increase in pain. With this success, she was able to determine the time and positioning requirements for the other tasks she wanted to accomplish.

Working Outside the Home

If you are considering a return to work or are still working, be sure you stick to a routine that includes taking care of yourself. Regular sleep, exercise, good nutrition, and stress management are good for everyone's health. When you have chronic pain, these are especially important. They help maintain your capacity to work, as do continued pacing, adaptation, and delegation.

Many people complain that pacing themselves at home is all well and good, but at work, "it's impossible!" Actually, you can use the same strategies in the workplace environment. It just takes a little more creative problem solving. For one thing, there are external time pressures at work; for another, pacing yourself in the workplace may involve synchronizing your work with that of other people. I generally recommend that you first identify the time and positioning requirements of your various work tasks. Next, create a diagram of how you can perform these tasks throughout the day using the pacing routine. This should include alternating between sitting and standing tasks, as well as between what you can do individually and what involves other people.

You can use sticky notes for each task, with its time and positioning requirements. Then move the notes around on a large piece of paper to help you organize your day.

Other strategies can include setting the timer on the computer and doing a minute of stretching every hour, or bringing a cot to lie on while listening at meetings. Or you may need to work with an occupational therapist to determine job modifications or the need for adaptive equipment. Again, let those around you know that you have specific needs. Telling them what works best for you allows you to assert choice. It also gives the clear message that you do not need to be rescued and that the situation is under control. There many be many people around you who would like to help but are at a loss as to what to do. Give them your guidelines; help them to help you and work with you more effectively.

Finally, I have had many patients realize that developing chronic pain gave them the opportunity to take another career path, one that allowed them to accommodate their new life with pain. They did so by returning to school or by taking technical training, by pursuing their more artistic and creative side, or by becoming self-employed. The key is being open to the possibilities, both old and new. Try this exercise to begin getting in touch with the possibilities.

Make a list of the skills, interests, and dreams you have. Brainstorm with friends and family members. If you get stuck go to *www.amazon.com* and plug "career change" into the "Book" query box. You will find that there are many books written on the topic and you may be able to find one that helps get you unstuck. Then ask yourself these questions.

> What interests me the most?
>
> What am I the best at or what would I like to become better at?
>
> What is my most passionate dream?

Is there a theme here? Can you combine your answers to these three questions (or to others) to form a starting point? Do a reality check to make sure that any new ideas can be worked with in pain, or identify how you might have to change them to acknowledge the pain. Then start making a list of steps to take to accomplish this goal. Sound familiar? Then get started on your fact-finding mission!

Common Problems When Becoming Active

If you find yourself needing hours or a whole day to recover from activities, you have probably not stopped an activity soon enough. You need to practice responding earlier to increases in tightness, fatigue, and pain. Your pain diary will help you fine-tune your pain sensation awareness, as will some exercises described later in this chapter.

Do you find yourself experiencing delayed pain increases? For example, you clean out the garage one day without excessive pain, but the next day you ache all over even more than before. If so, then you are probably experiencing the effects of "deconditioning." Deconditioning is decreased muscle strength and endurance from not getting regular exercise. This is a common problem for patients with chronic pain. A regular exercise (conditioning) program may be of great value. It will allow you to increase your endurance and limit muscle fatigue. Such a program may involve walking, swimming, using a stationary bicycle or treadmill, or practicing tai chi or yoga (see "Aerobic Exercise," below). The choice, of course, depends on where you are having pain and what your physical limitations are.

Remember, too, that your level of pain may not *necessarily* correlate with your ability to function. Many people are able to increase their activity level without increasing their pain. Once you go through the normal, expectable soreness and tightness of starting an activity routine, you may find yourself in no more pain than you were before. The exercises described later in the chapter may help you to discriminate between these normal feelings and pain that is a caution signal. The value in all of this is that you may be able to become more active in spite of the pain and without fear of harming yourself. This fear keeps many people with chronic pain inactive.

Time Management

In order to pace, adapt, and delegate effectively, it's important to take a look at all that you do during the course of a day. That way you can see exactly how much time you spend on certain activities. Putting a routine schedule into your life can make you feel useful again. Getting up and going to bed at the same time also helps establish a natural body rhythm. Having your day planned can help you accomplish your tasks and insures that pacing is not an afterthought. You may also find it very helpful to prepare a backup plan in advance for managing those inevitable flare-up days (see Chapter 10). Even if you can't work outside the home, consider volunteering. You can apply the pacing activities described here to help you be successful and reap the good feelings associated with helping others.

The Time Pie

An exercise that is helpful in determining what you do during a day is to draw a pie chart or "time pie." Break up your 24-hour day into the time periods that your different activities require. In other words, make each activity a wedge in the time pie. For example, you may have wedges for sleeping, working on the job, meeting with friends, talking on the phone, reading, watching TV, doing housework, playing with the kids, and so on. This is a nice way to graphically display what really takes place each day—something most people rarely think about. If each day of your week is different, then make seven time pies; if your weekdays are different from your weekends, make two time pies—one for weekdays and one for weekends. Draw your pie(s) in the space provided on the following page.

Now draw a pie that you would find more acceptable, given your pain level and what you are learning from this book. Ask yourself the following questions, and write down your answers:

1. How many hours of my day are devoted to meeting others' needs? _____

2. Do all of these activities really need my involvement? _____

3. What activities can I share with or assign to the person or persons who are currently requiring my time? _____

4. What activities that I am not currently pursuing would I like to add to (or put back into) my routine? _____

5. What steps can I take to make my present time pie into a more acceptable pie? _____

   _____

   _____

Use this space to draw your time pies—both your current one(s) and your ideal one:

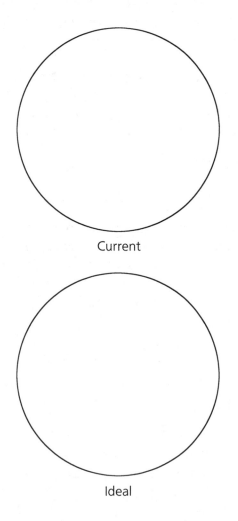

Current

Ideal

True Confessions: Choosing Your Activities Consciously

Most people get their sense of personal worth from the things they do. Which of your activities most define you? This is important to know because it affects how you plan activities and manage your time. For example, you may find it very difficult not to do all the tasks for your family. Altruism is ennobling, but it's not healthy for you (or for others) if you help others mindlessly or with secret bitterness. Helping mindlessly can lead to overdoing and hurting yourself. Doing for others because you feel you "have to" can create resentment and feelings of being used and abused. I'll never forget one patient who complained about how she had to get up early every morning to pack lunches for her children. When I inquired about their ages, thinking that if they were teenagers they might be old enough to pack their own lunches, she replied, "Oh, they're 26 and 28 years old!"

Another point you may wish to consider is this. People can use pain as an excuse not to do things they don't want to do. People can also use pain to control others and get attention they might not otherwise get. Sometimes people in chronic pain feel guilty when they become aware of such behaviors in themselves. I find that such behaviors are usually unconscious; they are the result of pain's effectiveness in both obtaining attention and avoiding undesirable obligations. Understanding how you incorporate your pain experience into your life can help you choose which behaviors you may want to develop further or avoid.

You really do have choices. This is your opportunity to explore a new you. It's okay to say "no." It's okay to say "yes." For now, it's enough that you make all of your choices conscious. If you choose to continue a certain activity or behavior, do it with your commitment and *your* choice: Own it.

Listening to Your Body

As noted at the beginning of this chapter, your body can be the source of important cues. By becoming aware of your body's messages, you can avoid problems and even soothe yourself. This section presents a series of exercises in learning to listen to your body. Read through the exercises once, then try them.

These exercises will help you do or learn the following:

- Gently stretch your muscles.
- Gently move your limbs through their range of motion.
- Isolate muscle tension.
- Relabel sensations.
- Use breathing to release tension.
- Develop body awareness.
- Experience the pleasant, energizing feelings that come from simple exercise.

If your muscles are not stretched and your limbs do not go through their range of motion, then your stiffness, tightness, and tension will increase, especially upon rising in the morning. If you limit your "exercise" to the movement involved in your daily chores, you will be likely to overextend and hurt tight muscles. Doing slow, purposeful exercises, such as the ones explained here, will help minimize injury.

If any of the following movements increases your pain, you can modify it so that a gentle stretch has no increase in pain. If you are unable to stretch a limb gently, then skip it (or imagine yourself doing the stretch in your mind) and go on to the next limb.

Labeling Sensations in Your Legs

1. Sit comfortably in a chair.

2. Point your right foot in front of you and lift it off the ground. Keep breathing slowly and regularly. How would you describe the sensation you feel? Tightness, stretching, burning, aching? (Avoid using the word "pain" or "it hurts"; these terms are too vague. Learning to describe the sensation more accurately may give you clues as to its cause and effect. This may lead to more specific remedies.) Also, where exactly do you feel these sensations? Front of lower leg, across the top of the foot, around the knee?

3. Now, as you point your right foot, become aware of the tension you may have placed in your left leg, arms, or face as you create the stretch. Make sure that only the right leg is tense, and relax the other parts of your body. Keep breathing slowly and regularly.

4. Take a deep breath. On the out-breath, release the tension in your right leg, letting the foot rest once again on the floor.

5. Close your eyes. How does your right leg feel compared with the left leg? Warm, tingling, tired, vibrant?

6. Now point your left foot in front of you and lift it off the ground. Make sure you don't get your arms or face involved in creating the tension, and keep breathing regularly. What sensations do you feel? Tightness, stretching, burning, aching?

7. Take a deep breath. On the out-breath, release the tension in your left leg, letting the foot rest once again on the floor.

8. Close your eyes and compare how your right and left legs feel now.

Labeling Sensations in Your Arms

While exercising your arms, make sure that your legs and face are not involved in the tension. And, once again, be sure to keep breathing slowly and regularly.

1. Make a fist with your right hand and hold your right arm out in front of you. How would you describe the sensations you feel? Where do you feel them?

2. Take a deep breath. On the out-breath, relax your fist and let the tension go, bringing your arm back down to your legs. How does your right arm feel compared with the left one?

3. Now make a fist with your left hand and hold your left arm out in front of you. What sensations do you feel? Where do you feel them?

4. Take a deep breath. On the out-breath, relax your fist and let the tension go, returning your arm to your lap. How does your left arm feel compared with the right one?

Labeling Sensations in Your Shoulders

Like the other exercises, this exercise should be done slowly, accompanied by nice, deep breaths.

1. Put the fingertips from both hands on their respective shoulders.

2. Raise your elbows out from your sides, and rotate the elbows as if you are drawing circles in the air.

3. Move your elbows in circles with each breath, so that each complete circle takes one slow breath. Make sure that the tension is only in your shoulders and upper back.

4. Draw circles in one direction five times, then draw circles in the other direction five times.

5. Take a deep breath. On the out-breath, let your hands fall gently back into your lap.

6. Close your eyes and see whether you can distinguish any sensation (tired, achy, vibrant, burning?) in your upper back, shoulders, and neck.

Labeling Sensations in Your Face

As in the previous exercises, breathing is very important; however, it may be a bit more difficult in this case because of the facial movements involved.

1. Imagine that you have just bitten into a lemon, and wrinkle your face.

2. Feel the tension in your face, and check to see whether the rest of your body is relaxed.

3. Keep breathing slowly and regularly. (This may be hard to do through a wrinkled nose!)

4. Take a deep breath. On the out-breath, relax your face.

5. Close your eyes. Now check out your whole body by doing a "body sweep."

That is, use your mind like a flashlight and shine it on each part of your body that you have just stretched. Release any residual tension by breathing into the tense area and breathing out the tension. How do you feel?

Rating Your Pain

The following exercise will help you to translate physical sensation into numbers. You may find this especially helpful if you have had any difficulty in giving your pain a numerical rating in your pain diary. You will use a scale of 0 to 10 for rating sensation in making fists, with 0 being the loosest fist and 10 being the tightest fist. Read through to the end of these instructions, and then do the exercise before you continue.

1. Make a number 5 fist. How would you describe the sensations you feel? Where do you feel them?

2. Relax the fist.

3. Now make a number 2 fist. What sensations do you feel? Where do you feel them? What makes the number 2 fist different from the number 5 fist?

4. Relax the fist.

5. Now make a number 9 fist. What sensations do you feel? Where do you feel them? What makes the number 9 fist different from the number 5 fist?

6. Relax the fist.

Be sure to try this exercise before you read on.

The following are some comments made by patients who did this exercise:

"Sensation is relative, and so is pain."

"A number 2 pain is more tolerable than a number 5 pain, but even a number 5 pain is tolerable compared to a number 9 pain."

"A number 2 pain is more localized, with the pain spreading away from the original painful area as the rating goes higher. . . . The higher the number given the pain, the more dysfunction is associated with it, both physically and emotionally."

When pain spreads it is often because of the added tension of holding your breath in response to pain. Remember the first breath-focusing exercise in Chapter 3 (the fist–breath exercise)? The pain sensation focuses your attention on the point in pain. This in turn increases your awareness of the pain, which increases your distress, which increases the muscle tension, and so on. Instead, you can take a deep breath and breathe out slowly.

Apply this to your own pain rating. See whether you can discern the subtleties of your sensations. What you once thought to be only one sensation may in fact be many. Develop an awareness of the muscle tension that comes from holding your breath or breathing shallowly. Can you identify the normal sensations of tightness and "good hurts" that are part of beginning an exercise routine? Continued practice with an RR technique will also help fine-tune this awareness. When you can distinguish these sensations, you will be better able to do activities and exercises safely. Even if these simple sensation-labeling exercises are all you can do on a regular basis, they will help keep your muscles, bones, and joints healthy.

Using Your Body to Change Your Mood

People communicate in many ways that have nothing to do with their words. My patients sometimes confide that they no longer tell their friends or family members when they are having a bad day. But they tell me this as they sit with their shoulders sagging and brows tense. They grimace as they frequently change positions, and they sigh a lot. Who's kidding whom?

These subtle behaviors are definite communications with the outside world. Sometimes the outside world is listening. But sometimes not being direct allows others to ignore you or to interpret your actions incorrectly. Most people cannot imagine living with chronic pain. When your body and your words give mixed messages, confusion results for you and for those watching you. Plus, when you assume body postures and facial expressions like the ones just described, you may be reinforcing negative emotions and making your situation even worse than it already is.

Try this simple exercise:

1. Raise your eyebrows and show your teeth.

2. Hold this posture for 30 seconds. What kinds of thoughts pass through your mind? (Ignore the ones that say you must look goofy.)

3. Relax.

4. Now bring your eyebrows together and clench your jaw and fists. What are you thinking now?

The first expression is usually associated with happiness, and the second one with anger and rage. How did you feel? Psychologist Paul Ekman and his colleagues (see "Supplementary Reading") have shown that assuming the facial expression that matches a specific emotion—such as happiness or anger—can produce the physiological changes linked to that emotion. When more of your body gets involved in the expression, the emotional connection is even greater.

Now for the final exercise in this chapter. This may be a bit uncomfortable for you, but it is important and helps you get in touch with your body–mind connection. If the sitting position is too difficult you can do the exercise lying on your bed in a fetal position—knees to chest, head down toward chest.

1. Sit in a chair.

2. Bend your head down, hunch your shoulders, cross your arms in front of you, and cross your legs.

3. Close your eyes for one minute. What do you *feel* emotionally? Do not use the word "pain," and stick to descriptions of emotions, not descriptions of physical sensations.

4. Relax.

5. Now stand up and place your feet apart, approximately the width of your hips.

6. Keep your shoulders back, your head up, your face to the front, and your arms down with the palms facing forward.

7. Close your eyes. What do you *feel* now?

The first position is associated with a wide range of feelings, such as the following:

- Sadness
- Fear
- Defenselessness
- Need for safety
- Need for security

The second position is usually associated with these feelings:

- Empowerment
- Being exposed
- Sense of control
- Positive attitude

Your emotional responses to body posture reflect a complex body–mind language that you have learned automatically over the years. This is why people will sometimes experience strong emotional reactions during massage therapy or certain physical therapy procedures. This muscular imprinting of emotions and old habits is also the principle behind various movement therapies, in particular, Feldenkrais and the Alexander technique.

When you are feeling sad, try to change your facial expression and body posture to those associated with joy and happiness. See how difficult it is to continue feeling sad. Or, if you're committed to suffering for the moment, exaggerate your suffering expression and posture even more. Don't forget to add a few moans. If you do this consciously, you may be surprised at the results. Misery loves company, even if it's your own.

Aerobic Exercise

Moderate aerobic exercise at least 30 minutes a day, 5 days or more a week can help improve your general health, particularly your heart and lung function. It can also help with weight control at 60 minutes a day and weight loss at 90 minutes a day. Aerobic exercise ("aerobic" means literally "requires oxygen") elevates heart rate through sustained movements of the body at moderate intensity. Activities such as brisk walking, swimming, and stationary bicycling are considered aerobic exercise. There is a long list of diseases associated with a sedentary lifestyle—for example, heart disease, obesity, and osteoporosis. The risk of developing these disorders can be reduced by regular aerobic exercise. Just because you're in pain doesn't mean you need to neglect your overall health and well-being. Quite the contrary, in fact.

Physiatrist James Rainville and others have found that pain perception and the ability to be active do not always match, particularly in patients with low back pain. This is probably because most perceptions are subjective. A lot of people who have pain are afraid to move because they fear they will harm themselves further and increase the pain. But by not moving, and by not stretching or exercising, they become even more out of shape and more at risk for reinjury. Regular exercise may also be effective in reducing your pain, as demonstrated in arthritis patients (see Minor and Sanford in "Supplementary Reading"). If you exercise carefully and slowly, you are not likely to make your condition worse. Consult your physician or a physical therapist if you have specific questions regarding what you can do and how you should proceed. Those of you with low back pain may find the physical activity and exercise descriptions in *The Back Pain Helpbook* beneficial (see "Supplementary Reading").

For people in pain, water exercises can be especially relaxing, because about 70% of the effects of gravity are lost in water. Movement in water offers the opportunity to strengthen muscles, stretch, and increase heart and lung function. The Arthritis Foundation sponsors water aerobics programs all across the United States. Contact the Arthritis Foundation in your state for details. Since movement is so much easier in water, however, you may be tempted to exercise longer and harder. It's always best to start out doing much less than you think you can do and gradually increase the length or intensity of your water exercise as you progress.

Other forms of exercise that can give you a good aerobic workout include the following:

- Riding a stationary bike.
- Walking on a treadmill.
- Using indoor cross-country ski equipment.
- Walking. (This is a particularly good exercise, as it's inexpensive and can be done almost anywhere, indoors or outdoors.)
- Yoga or tai chi. (These exercises are helpful to patients in pain because they are slow, purposeful, and coordinated with breathing. They can also be easily adapted for those with limited movement. It is important, however, to get individual instruction and work with an instructor who can modify the positions to meet your needs.)

My colleagues and I strongly encourage people in chronic pain to do some type of aerobic, stretching, and strengthening exercise on a regular basis. If at all possible, do this for the health of both your body and mind.

Pleasurable Activities

Little Things

Most of us miss out
on life's big prizes.
The Pulitzer. The Nobel. Oscars. Tonys. Emmys.
But we're all eligible for
life's small pleasures.
A pat on the back.
A kiss
behind the ear.
A four-pound bass.
A full moon.
An empty parking space.
A crackling fire. A great meal. A glorious sunset.
Hot soup.
Cold beer.
Don't fret about copping life's grand awards.
Enjoy its tiny delights.
There are plenty for all of us.

—*Anonymous*

Pleasurable activities should constitute a normal part of life, but for many living with chronic pain, they simply don't. Some patients feel so bad about their pain and their lack of a "productive life" that they cannot engage in pleasurable activities or even admit they want to. They feel that they don't deserve any pleasure.

The truth of the matter is that if you can't do some pleasurable things, it will be difficult to increase your activities in general. It's easier to start becoming involved in life again by doing something that gives you pleasure. (See the book *Healthy Pleasures* in the "Supplementary Reading" section at the end of this chapter.)

There are any number of ways to pursue pleasurable activities, but let's just say that you should do something purposeful, conscious, and enjoyable on a regular basis. It can be as simple as feeding the birds, watching the sunset, or observing children at play. It doesn't have to be an outing, though it can be. It's often the little things in life that make our days meaningful. The key here is to make it *conscious and purposeful*. As the philosopher Epictetus (circa A.D. 55–135) said, "Practice yourself, for heaven's sake, in little things; and thence proceed to greater." In addition, take an active part in creating your own happiness. Doing something that is someone else's idea of a pleasurable activity doesn't count unless you truly take pleasure from that person's enjoyment. Also, when you have completed your pleasurable activity, don't spend 10 minutes describing how miserable you were and apologizing for engaging in it. There is something to be said for counting your blessings.

It's possible that you may be intimidated by having to seek out a pleasurable activity. Substituting the word "satisfaction" or "beauty" for "pleasure" helps. Look for something that you can feel satisfied with or that has a beauty you can identify.

Once you have discovered and enjoyed a pleasurable activity, try sharing it with someone. For example, if you just saw a beautiful sunrise on your way to work, you could share it with a colleague. People, it seems, are always willing to give a litany of their disappointments, but it is amazing how uplifting the sharing of pleasures can be. It's also a lovely way to begin dinner conversation. Let everyone have a turn to report a little pleasure they noted that day. Life has a whole different feel to it when you become an active participant.

In short, it's okay to do something nice and pleasurable for yourself. You're worth it!

Summary

Increasing Activities

- You can keep active while in pain by using pacing, adaptation, and delegation.

- When the body is not in a constant state of exhaustion, it has a chance to recover more effectively.

Time Management

- Drawing a "time pie" helps you identify your daily activities and the time spent on them; it provides you with a picture of how you spend each day.

- Take a look at each activity, and examine why you engage in it.

- Consider asking for assistance from others who are capable of helping.

Listening to Your Body

- Listen to your body and label your sensations. Developing an awareness of your body allows you to increase activity safely. It also lets you stop growing muscle tension earlier than you otherwise would.

- Try gentle stretching exercises that move your limbs through their range of motion. This will also help you to label sensations in various parts of your body.

- The exercises also help relieve the stress, tension, and stiffness usually associated with inactivity.

- Learn not to label all body sensations as painful. Distinguishing pain from other sensations will help you to pace activities, such as exercise, more realistically.

Using Your Body to Change Your Mood

- Your body posture and facial expression can either bring your emotions down further or lift your spirits.
- Pay attention to how your body is communicating with the outside world as well as with your internal world; you have the power to change how you feel.

Aerobic Exercise

- Aerobic exercise at least five times a week can help improve your general health, particularly your heart and lung function; it can also help with weight control.
- Water exercises are particularly helpful, because about 70% of the effects of gravity are lost in water.
- Other types of exercise that can give you a good workout include the following:
  —Riding a stationary bike
  —Walking on a treadmill
  —Using indoor cross-country ski equipment
  —Walking
  —Yoga or tai chi

Pleasurable Activities

- Pleasurable activities should be conscious and purposeful. They help you become more involved in life and make your days meaningful.
- Once you have discovered a pleasurable activity, share it with someone.
- You deserve to engage in pleasurable activities for your psychological and physical health.

Exploration Tasks

1. Reread this chapter and do the various exercises as they are presented, if you have not already done so.

2. Write out a goal that you want to accomplish related to this chapter. As in earlier goal-setting exercises, make sure your goal is a behavioral task that you can measure in terms of the steps that *you* will take to accomplish it. Here is an example:

Goal: <u>Do the stretches described in the section "Listening to Your Body" once a</u> <u>day.</u>

Steps to take to reach that goal:

A. <u>Use the kitchen chair.</u>

B. <u>Place the instructions on a second chair beside me.</u>

C. <u>Do the stretches just before I do my RR technique.</u>

Now it's your turn.

Goal: _____

Steps to take to reach that goal:

A. _____

B. _____

C. _____

D. _____

Now list contingency plans. That is, identify what obstacles might get in the way of your accomplishing this goal. What solutions can you devise to work toward insuring the success of this goal? See Chapter 3 ("The Mind–Body Connection") for an explanation of contingency plans if you've forgotten what they are and why they're useful.

Obstacles	**Solutions**
A. _____	_____
B. _____	_____
C. _____	_____
D. _____	_____

3. Identify some type of stretching exercise that you can do daily. What will you do? How often will you be able to do it? _____

4. Identify some type of aerobic exercise that you can do at least five times a week. What will you do? _____

   How often will you be able to do it? _____

5. Identify some type of strengthening program that you can do three times per week. This can involve isometrics with an elasticized cord for that purpose, free weights, or weight machines. A good resource for women (and men) is *Strong Women Stay Young* and *Strong Women and Men Beat Arthritis* (see "Supplementary Reading"). Ask your medical professional for recommendations or a physical therapy referral for a safe exercise program you can do that takes all your physical limitations (not only your pain) into consideration.

What will you do? _____

How often will you be able to do it? _____

6. Continue with one of the basic RR techniques (see Chapter 3) at least once a day.

7. Choose a pleasurable activity and engage in it once a week at a minimum. Share it with someone.

List some pleasurable activities that you might like to try:

_____

_____

_____

_____

(Don't forget the spontaneous pleasures, like listening to children's laughter or reveling in a sunny day.)

8. If your pain increases with certain activities or postures during your daily routine, take some time to fill out the "Increasing Activities Worksheet" at the end of this book. Determine your average daily level of pain from your daily diary sheet as your baseline pain.

Now make a list of activities that increase and decrease your pain. What are the common threads identifying each category? Posture? Length of time? Fatigue? Motivation? What happens if you alternate the activities that increase pain with those that decrease pain? Can you fine-tune any of the activities to make them easier to do in bits, like John did (for example, dividing the laundry to carry downstairs into four smaller bundles)?

Remember, the goal is to keep active while not significantly increasing the pain. This takes changes in your daily routine, but a lot can still be accomplished.

Beware of telling yourself, "Just one more dish [minute, task, etc.] before stopping." Use external cues such as timers to dictate when the time is up and/or your position needs to be changed.

As you continue working with the entire program, you will need to reassess your routine periodically, because your endurance may increase as your tension decreases. Make copies of the Increasing Activities Worksheet at the back of the book so that you can reassess your progress periodically.

Supplementary Reading

The following books and articles provide additional information on exercise, body awareness, and healthy pleasures:

Lorna Bell and Eudora Seyfer, *Gentle Yoga* (Berkeley, CA: Celestial Arts, 1987).

Paul Ekman, Robert Levenson, and Wallace Friesen, "Autonomic Nervous System Activity Distinguishes among Emotions," *Science, 221*: 1208–1210, 1983.

John Gormley and Juliette Hussey (Eds.), *Exercise Therapy: Prevention and Treatment of Disease* (Malden, MA: Blackwell, 2005).

Carol Krucoff, Mitchell Krucoff, and Adam Brill, *Healing Moves: How to Cure, Relieve, and Prevent Common Ailments with Exercise* (New York: Crown Publishers, 2000).

Kate Lorig and James Fries, *The Arthritis Helpbook: A Tested Self-Management Program for Coping with Arthritis and Fibromyalgia, Sixth Edition* (New York: Da Capo Press, 2006).

M. A. Minor and M. K. Sanford, "Physical Interventions in the Management of Pain in Arthritis," *Arthritis Care and Research, 6*: 197–206, 1993.

James Moore, Kate Lorig, Michael VanKorff, Virginia Gonzalez, and Diane Laurent, *The Back Pain Helpbook* (Reading, MA: Perseus Books, 1999).

Miriam Nelson, Kristin Baker, and Ronenn Roubenoff, with Lawrence Lindner, *Strong Women and Men Beat Arthritis* (New York: G. P. Putnam's Sons, 2002).

Miriam Nelson, Wendy Wray, and Sarah Wernick, *Strong Women Stay Young* (New York: Bantam, 2005).

Robert Ornstein and David Sobel, *Healthy Pleasures* (New York: Da Capo Press, 1990).

James Rainville, David Ahern, Linda Phalen, Lisa Childs, and Robin Sutherland, "The Association of Pain with Physical Activities in Chronic Low Back Pain," *Spine, 17*: 1060–1064, 1992.

U.S. Department of Health and Human Services, Centers for Disease Control and Prevention, National Center for Chronic Disease Prevention and President's Council on Physical Fitness, *Physical Activity and Health: A Report of the Surgeon General* (Sudbury, MA: Jones and Bartlett, 1998).

5

The Power of the Mind

My anxiety stems from a feeling that no one is there to take
care of me. If I give in to the pain, react the way I really feel,
my world will fall apart, I won't have any income, my
husband will leave, no one will like me. I am worried all the
time about getting things done, screwing things up, letting
others down, making other people angry. I need to escape. I
need to be released from these worries by having someone say:
"Start over. Build a life based on what you want, and let the
other chips fall where they may." If I did that, what if I
couldn't figure out what I wanted? What if I was still unhappy
and without a husband, job, or money?
— *Passage from a writing exercise on pain by Joan, a patient*

Harnessing the Power of the Mind: Cognitive Techniques

We know that certain ways of thinking—for example, catastrophizing, denial,
avoidance, and wishful thinking—are associated with disability in chronic pain.
Much of this thinking has to do with feeling out of control. We also know that
thinking patterns can be changed to make you feel more in control. That is why I
strongly encourage you to take the following pages to heart.

People who catastrophize tend to exaggerate disappointments and negative
events ("This is the worst thing that could happen to me. I'll never get better"). Denial allows people to ignore their need to pace activities ("Nothing is wrong with
me"). Avoidance of social events can isolate; avoidance of movement can weaken
muscles ("If I don't move at all, I'll be all right"). Wishful thinking can make a person postpone getting help for pain management ("I'll just wait. Maybe my pain will
be gone soon.")

We know from research that people with certain beliefs about pain—for example, "The pain is mysterious and unknowable," "What happens to me is determined
by chance," or "Whatever happens to me is out of my control and will defeat
me"—tend to have more negative emotions and disability. This is why it's impor-

tant for you to have information about pain that makes it all less mysterious. It is also why a healthy approach to treatment includes exploration of your thoughts, feelings, and beliefs. This exploration can take advantage of the complex mind–body experience of pain. It can also help repair damaged self-esteem and help you gain control over your pain.

The mind, the source of thoughts and feelings, gives meaning to our experiences, including pain. If you are in a self-defeated, hopeless frame of mind, you will most likely interpret pain signals in a negative way, increasing distress and despair. The mind is like a filter; the pain signal passes through it and is either dampened or magnified. On a warm, sunny day, or when someone has said "I love you," or when you have received a letter from a friend you've been missing, your pain experience may not be as grim as it is on a cold, rainy day when no one has called you in weeks and you have nothing to do.

You have already begun to harness the power of the mind with your practice of the RR techniques (see Chapter 3). The work described in this chapter will ask you to explore some of the things that determine how you see the world around you. The techniques presented here are called cognitive techniques. "Cognitive" comes from "cognition," which means "knowing" or "thinking." To begin, let's look at the content of what you think and how that influences your emotions.

Self-Talk or Automatic Thoughts

Listen to what you say to yourself as you react to situations. We call this "self-talk." Many emotions are kept going, if not created, by self-talk. If you change the way you talk to yourself, you can actually change how you feel.

For example, reread the passage from Joan's writing exercise presented at the beginning of this chapter. What do your feel? Do you sense the panic, anxiety, and fear that she felt just by reading her written thoughts? If you do, it shows you the power of thoughts. If you find yourself judging the content instead, you may benefit from reading the section on empathy in the next chapter.

Self-talk can go with positive as well as negative emotions. Some people are thought to routinely practice positive self-talk (the optimists); others go through a daily torrent of negative thoughts (the pessimists). The following excerpt from *The Subtleties of the Inimitable Mulla Nasrudin,* a collection of Middle Eastern tales by Idries Shah, demonstrates the point.

I Only Hope I'm Ill

Nasrudin came late among the crowd waiting for the doctor's attentions. He was repeating in a loud voice, over and over again: "I hope I'm very ill, I hope I'm very ill." He so demoralized the other sufferers that they insisted on his going in to see the physician first.

"I only hope I'm very ill!"

"Why?"

"I'd hate to think that anyone who feels like me was really fit and well!" (p. 78)

For obvious reasons, you will want to address the self-talk that is negative. You already feel bad enough, and sustained negative emotions take the joy out of living. They also add to feelings of helplessness and hopelessness and can increase disability.

Self-talk is automatic, happens very quickly, and doesn't always come in complete sentences. For example, let's suppose that you wake up in the morning and open your eyes. You make your first attempt to get out of bed and you become aware of the pain. You might say to yourself: "It's still here. Ugh! I can't stand it anymore! When will it go away? I've suffered enough. I'm useless! I'll never get better. This is going to be a miserable day. Life is miserable. I'm miserable. No one cares." If you talk to yourself like this, why *wouldn't* you feel sad or despondent?

But be careful not to confuse negative thinking with judging thoughts as "bad"—or "good." The issue is not whether they are good or bad, but whether they are helpful or unhelpful.

We all engage in negative self-talk at one time or another. However, much negative self-talk is inaccurate. It can distort events in ways that make us feel defeated and helpless. In the "getting out of bed" example, the self-talk about pain is depressing and anxiety provoking because it combines both realistic and unrealistic descriptions. It's true that the pain is still there and you're miserable. However, the other statements are exaggerated, black-and-white assumptions whose accuracy can and should be challenged. You aren't necessarily useless because you have pain, and you really don't know whether the *whole* day will be miserable, and, in any event, what's that got to do with people caring about you?

There is power in cognitive work; it gives you the opportunity to challenge what you say to yourself. Is what you say to yourself accurate? Are there other ways to look at your situation? A passage from *The Pleasantries of the Incredible Mulla Nasrudin,* another of Idries Shah's books, illustrates this:

I Believe You Are Right!

The Mulla was made magistrate. During his first case, the plaintiff argued so persuasively that [Nasrudin] exclaimed: "I believe that you are right!" The clerk of the court begged him to restrain himself, for the defendant had not been heard yet.

Nasrudin was so carried away by the eloquence of the defendant that he cried out as soon as the man had finished his evidence: "I believe you are right!" The clerk of the court could not allow this.

"Your honor, they cannot *both* be right."

"I believe you are right!" said Nasrudin. (p. 48)

Suppose that you are driving to an appointment and get caught in traffic. Let's imagine two different ways you could respond:

Response Set 1

The thoughts: "I can't believe this is happening to me! Where did all these people come from? Don't they know I have an important appointment? I'll never make it on time. This always happens to me. I should have known the traffic would be heavy. I'm so stupid. What a jerk!"

Physical response: Increased blood pressure and heart rate; short, shallow breathing; increased muscle tension . . . in short, the stress response.

Emotional response: Anger, frustration, and guilt.

Response Set 2

The thoughts: "What a drag. This is very unfortunate. My options to get out of this traffic jam are limited because I'm on a bridge. I may be late, but I can't control that right now. I'll use this opportunity to practice some diaphragmatic breathing while I put my favorite Mozart tape in the tape deck. I'll take a mini-vacation!"

Physical response: If anything, a decrease in blood pressure and heart rate; slowed breathing; decreased muscle tension.

Emotional response: Resolution, acceptance, and control.

What are the differences in the two sets of responses? What is it in the nature of the thoughts in Response Set 1 that might make you angry and frustrated? Underline the statements in Response Set 1 that are an accurate description of the situation. Now consider Response Set 2: How is it different from Response Set 1? Underline the statements in Response Set 2 that accurately describe the situation.

Your immediate reaction to all of this may be that you have a right to get agitated and frustrated when bad things happen. You certainly do! But we are talking about choices. If getting aggravated and agitated is your choice, go right ahead. However, if negative emotions increase your physical pain, then read on.

Irrational and Distorted Thoughts

Where do these "wild and crazy" thoughts come from? Why are they sometimes such distortions of what is really going on? Modern psychology and research on consciousness are only now beginning to appreciate the potential of the mind and the need for all of us to understand how and why we think the way we do.

The following observations (see "Supplementary Reading") may stimulate you to begin your own journey toward greater awareness of your thinking processes:

- Our cultural beliefs and vocabulary influence what we perceive of the world around us (Edward Hall and Robert Cialdini).

- Our predisposition for short-term planning leaves us vulnerable to long-term consequences (Robert Ornstein).

- Gender, as well as culture, influences our interpersonal communication (Deborah Tannen).

A good place to start is to identify the content of the assumptions and beliefs that lie behind your self-talk. Psychologists and other thinkers have made several attempts at identifying the sources of negative thoughts, and these ideas are not necessarily new.

> Men are disturbed not by things which happen, but by the opinions about the things. . . . When we are impeded or disturbed or grieved, let us never blame others, but ourselves, that is our opinion. It is the act of an ill-instructed man to blame others for his bad condition; it is the act of one who has begun to be instructed, to lay the blame on himself; and of one whose instruction is completed, neither to blame another, nor himself. (Epictetus, circa A.D. 55–135, *The Encheiridion*)

Ellis's Irrational Beliefs

Psychologist Albert Ellis has developed a way to challenge exaggerated thoughts and replace them with more realistic ones. Called "rational–emotive therapy," it is based on the idea that much of our suffering comes from the irrational ways we think about the world. Self-defeating thoughts limit our possibilities. Here is a list of Ellis's ten "irrational beliefs" (from Ellis; see "Supplementary Reading"). I like to call them "the assumptions and beliefs that get us into trouble."

1. It is an absolute necessity for an adult to have love and approval from peers, family, and friends.

2. You must be unfailingly competent and almost perfect in all you undertake.

3. Certain people are evil, wicked, and villainous and should be punished.

4. It is horrible when people and things are not the way you would like them to be.

5. External events cause most human misery—people simply react as events trigger their emotions.

6. You should feel fear or anxiety about anything that is unknown, uncertain, or potentially dangerous.

7. It is easier to avoid than to face life's difficulties and responsibilities.

8. You need something other or stronger or greater than yourself to rely on.

9. The past has a lot to do with determining the present.

10. Happiness can be achieved by inaction, passivity, and endless leisure.

These beliefs are not *necessarily* irrational or crazy. That is, they are not absolutely untrue under all circumstances. But they are certainly irrational if you believe they are absolutely true under all circumstances, For example, making mistakes does feel horrible, but it is also part of being human. The lesson is to learn from them.

The Nature of "Truth"

Your first response after reading the list of Ellis's irrational beliefs may be this: "But how can these be irrational? They are all true!" If so, take a moment to think about the nature of "truth."

I'll never forget talking to a group of patients about being passed in the breakdown lane as they sat stuck in a traffic jam. The condemnations poured out: "They have no right to do that." "They're creeps." "Where are the police when you need them?" I then asked how many had *never* driven in the breakdown lane on that road. Nobody raised a hand.

We get caught up in the "truth" sometimes, but whose "truth" are we talking about? A passage from a third Idries Shah collection, *The Exploits of the Incomparable Mulla Nasrudin,* illustrates that this can be a tricky question:

How Nasrudin Created Truth

"Laws as such do not make people better," said Nasrudin to the King. "They must practice certain things in order to become attuned to inner truth. This *form* of truth resembles apparent truth only slightly."

The King decided that he could, and would, make people observe the truth. He could make them practice truthfulness.

His city was entered by a bridge. On this he built a gallows. The following day, when the gates were opened at dawn, the Captain of the Guard was stationed with a squad of troops to examine all who entered.

An announcement was made: "Everyone will be questioned. If he tells the truth, he will be allowed to enter. If he lies, he will be hanged."

Nasrudin stepped forward.

"Where are you going?"

"I am on my way," said Nasrudin slowly, "to be hanged."

"We don't believe you!"

"Very well, if I have told a lie, hang me!"

"But if we hang you for lying, we will have made what you said come true!"

"That's right; now you know what the truth is—YOUR truth!" (p. 7)

Burns's 10 Types of Cognitive Distortions

Another way of classifying negative self-talk comes from David Burns, a psychiatrist whose writings have brought cognitive techniques to a wider public. He found

10 common cognitive distortions that can cause problems. They also fuel catastrophic thinking. Read the following and see if some sound familiar to you:

1. *All-or-nothing thinking* (evaluating people or situations in extreme, black-or-white terms). For example, you used to play baseball on the weekends before you developed chronic pain. Now you find yourself thinking, "If I can't play baseball, I can't enjoy the sport anymore at all."

   There is an apparent advantage to thinking in all-or-nothing terms. It is more predictable and creates the feeling that there is order in the world around you. This, in turn, should give you an edge in controlling your world. Unfortunately, it doesn't work that way. Uncertainty is all that we have. Living comfortably with uncertainty is possible, but it takes time to master. The skills you are about to learn will help.

2. *Overgeneralization* (seeing a single negative event as a never-ending pattern of defeat). If you wake up in more pain, you might think, "I'll never be able to enjoy anything anymore." Globalizing misfortune in this way unnecessarily increases your misery.

3. *Mental filtering* (letting a single negative experience negatively color the whole situation). For example, you are preparing lunch for some friends and discover that you do not have an essential ingredient. All you can think about is how the whole lunch will be ruined. It gives you indigestion.

4. *Disqualifying the positive* (taking neutral or even positive experiences and turning them into negative ones). For example, a friend comes over to visit and tells you that you look great. Your immediate thought is this: "I don't feel great. She doesn't understand." Maybe not, but try a simple "thank you" first before you check it out. Maybe you don't look as bad as you feel!

5. *Jumping to conclusions* (quickly jumping to a negative conclusion that is not justified by the facts of the situation). Two types of jumping to conclusions are mind reading and fortune telling.

   A. *Mind reading.* You assume you know why someone else does what he or she does, and you don't bother to check it out. For example, you pass a coworker in the hallway and say "Hi!" He doesn't respond. You think, "He must be upset with me. What did I do wrong?" When you check it out, you find that the coworker was preoccupied about a sick child he had just left at home.

   B. *Fortune telling.* You "know" that things will turn out badly. You predict it as an established fact. For example, you wake up with a headache. You say, "Now my whole day is ruined. I had so much to do and I'll never get it all done."

6. *Magnification and minification.* In magnification, you exaggerate the importance of a negative event or mistake. For example, if you have a flareup in your pain, you say to yourself, "I can't stand this! I can't take this anymore!" As a matter of fact, however, you can. You may not want to, and that's okay, but you can take it. In minification, you take positive personal qualities or events and deny their importance. For example, a family member comments on how nice it is to see you at a family outing, and you reply, "A lot of good it does if I can't participate in the activities."

7. *Emotional reasoning* (taking your emotions as evidence for the truth). If you *feel* that something is right, then it must be true. For example, you find yourself thinking, "I feel useless. [Therefore] I *am* useless."

8. *Labeling* (identifying a mistake or negative quality and then describing an entire situation or individual in terms of that quality). For example, instead of seeing yourself as an individual who has a pain problem, you find yourself saying, "I'm defective, imperfect, and without any redeeming qualities."

9. *Personalization* (taking responsibility for a negative event even when the circumstances are beyond your control). For example, you and your spouse go out to eat at a fancy restaurant, but the service and food are poor. You find yourself feeling responsible for making a bad choice and "ruining" your evening together.

10. *"Should" statements* (attempts to motivate—or browbeat—yourself by saying things like "I should know better," "I should go there," or "I must do that"). Such statements set you up to feel resentful and pressured. They also imply that you are complying with an external authority.

Old "Tapes"

The irrational beliefs and cognitive distortions described above are old "tapes" that we play from our early experiences as children. They reflect our observations of our families, our teachers, and the larger society. Loretta Laroche, a comedian who teaches these principles through humor, conjures up a powerful image of a big yellow school bus that each person drives through life. Various people get on and off, but some have a lifetime ticket. They may include parents, teachers, ex-lovers, friends, and mentors, both alive and dead. There's always someone who thinks he or she knows the best way of getting where you're going, and sometimes that person will be found in the driver's seat. But this is your opportunity to decide who's really driving your bus. To return to the "tapes" metaphor, it's your opportunity to edit your old tapes and make some new ones.

There are different kinds of tapes with different recurring themes. For example, you either assume all the responsibility or none of it ("The pain is all my fault" or

"The pain is all your fault"). Or you expect a consistency in the world that doesn't exist ("If I'm good, bad things won't happen to me"). Or perhaps you feel that if you think negatively, it will ward off bad fortune ("I'm feeling better this morning, but if I tell anyone the pain might get worse"). Thinking in restricted, unconscious patterns (the old tapes) often robs you of the flexibility needed to cope with the ever-changing world and your personal problems.

Monitoring Self-Talk (Automatic Thoughts)

An Exercise Format

Because self-talk is so automatic, you need to catch it as happens. At the back of the book, there is a "Daily Record of Automatic Thoughts (Self-Talk)" worksheet that you can copy and carry with you. Each time you find yourself feeling sad, frustrated, or anxious, pull out the sheet to record your automatic thoughts and other responses. Tracking these thoughts will help you see what you've been saying to yourself and how that makes you feel. With this knowledge you can begin to act, rather than react, in response to events occurring around you. Again, don't judge the "goodness" or "badness" of negative thinking; that's not the point. The point is that thinking negatively for long periods is simply not helpful for problem solving.

So how should you record your self-talk? Here is an example:

Imagine that you wake up with increased pain on a day you had planned to visit a friend. (*Situation*)

What do you find yourself thinking? (*Automatic thoughts*) _____

How do you feel physically? (*Physical response*) _____

How do you feel emotionally? (*Emotional response*) _____

Do your thoughts match any of the cognitive distortions or irrational beliefs listed on the previous pages? (*Cognitive distortions*) _____

What is really going on and what action can you take? (*Changed thought,* to be discussed later) _____

I encourage you to carry the form with you because you can't always count on memory. Emotions and thoughts fade as time passes. Even in the moment, you may be aware only of physical symptoms, such as muscle tension or palpitations, and not emotions or thoughts. Just write down as much as you can about the situation and your physical sensations. That can help you recapture your emotions and thoughts. Slowly, with time and practice, you will be able to change negative responses as they occur. Remember, too, that you can use this exercise to explore your emotions and cognitions about anything, not just your pain.

Working with Anger

Anger is a powerful emotion and there are important reasons to control it. It has potential health risks (heart disease, substance abuse) and it can lead to social damage (road rage, sexual and physical abuse). Many people get angry in reaction to frustration or hurt. When someone or something has hurt you, the reaction triggered may be "fight," not "flight." This sets off a major adrenaline rush that can be difficult to control. Much of the work with self-talk is about changing the way you respond to events. But being angry can make such changes difficult. Angry people often blame others. That attitude can be a problem if you can't consider another point of view that acknowledges the harm done while accepting the need to move on with healing.

For many people, giving up their anger feels as though they are giving in to guilt for a pain problem that may clearly not be their fault. Assigning responsibility for an injury—the driver ran the red light and hit my car—can bring about legal resolution of wrongdoing. However, holding on to the anger about the wrongdoing makes you feel more victimized, depressed, and anxious. There are specific exercises that can help control anger, and you've already started doing many of them, including relaxation techniques. These exercises help you buy time between an event and your emotional response to it. Physical exercise helps check the stress effects of anger. The thinking skills that we've started to address in this chapter also help, as do journaling and the communication skills described later. Anger is discussed more fully in the next chapter. Other resources for anger management can be found in the "Supplementary Reading" section.

"Why Me?"

Sometimes you may think, "Why did this happen to me? When will it end? Why me? Why? Why? Why?" These questions can be overwhelming. You may think that you *should* be able to answer them. They give you the illusion that you are exploring and trying to solve problems. In fact, it's impossible to answer such questions.

Instead, take a look at the assumptions behind the questions. For example, do you feel that there is a reason for everything and that you should know it? Do you have a secret fear that anyone who feels this horrible must have done something pretty bad? If you were told that your pain would end in exactly 6 years and 2 months, would you be able to live comfortably now? Are these your assumptions? Do you have others? Compare them with the irrational beliefs and cognitive distortions described earlier. Which ones match your assumptions?

Don't confuse these "Why?" questions with the search for meaning in life. Meaning won't be found in an endless litany of "Why me?" In the end, such questions are just another form of negative and unhelpful thinking.

Changing Your Thoughts

> The greatest revolution of our time is the knowledge that
> human beings, by changing the inner attitudes of their minds,
> can transform the outer aspects of their lives.
>
> —*William James*

You can begin changing your self-talk by using one of three techniques.

Technique 1: Challenging Self-Talk (Automatic Thoughts)

In this first technique, you challenge the reality of your self-talk. First, capture your negative, automatic thoughts. You can use the worksheet mentioned earlier. Next, examine the captured thoughts for distortions, irrational beliefs, and self-defeating attitudes. With this groundwork in place, you can then challenge the accuracy of the thoughts. Often, after you challenge the thoughts, your emotional response will disappear.

For example, is it true that if you have chronic pain, you're defective and imperfect? By now, I would hope that you can respond with a loud "No!" What *is* true is this: You have a chronic problem that changes the way you do things. The statement "I'm defective" is a gross exaggeration. It's "labeling"—number 8 in Burns's list of cognitive distortions. Recognizing this, you may now be able to tell yourself: "Being in pain means I can do less but it does not reflect on my character" or "I can still accomplish things by pacing my activities; I show the courage to rise above my disability." How does that feel?

Be careful about one thing. Don't replace inaccurate negative thoughts with inaccurate positive ones. For example, when you wake up in pain, don't replace "My whole day is ruined" with "This is a wonderful experience." You will know when you hit on the right statement because you will feel better, relieved, less anxious, or less sad.

Using Technique 1, how might you change your self-talk on waking up with increased pain on a day you had made plans to visit a friend? Write your new self-talk here.

_____

_____

_____

Technique 2: Clarifying the Problem and What You Can Do

Here is a second way to change your self-talk. It helps you clarify the real problem and see where you have some control even in a seemingly impossible situation. Here are the steps, with an example:

State the problem: <u>I am awakening in pain.</u>

State why it's a problem: <u>Because I had plans to visit a friend today.</u>

Identify:

What can you do? <u>I will see how I feel after taking a hot shower, an RR technique, and taking two aspirin.</u>

What do you need? <u>I can ask that my friend come here, or that we meet somewhere closer. Or I can visit her another time. This happens. It is usually self-limited. I know what I can do to take care of myself.</u>

How do you feel? <u>Sad, but in control.</u>

Technique 3: The Vertical Arrow or "So What?" Technique

Sometimes your discouraging self-talk may seem so accurate that you have trouble seeing where the problem is. In these situations, try the vertical arrow technique, designed by David Burns (see "Supplementary Reading"). You begin by buying into the negative thought and asking yourself, "If what I'm saying to myself is true, then why does it upset me?" "So what?" Then ask yourself, "What's the worst that could happen?" You then write down your answer and draw an arrow pointing down from what you have written.

Next, you ask yourself the same questions, but this time about the answer you just wrote down. Under the arrow, you write down another answer, then draw another arrow. Ask yourself the questions again. You continue until you have gone as far as you can. This should uncover all the cognitive distortions, irrational beliefs, fears, and assumptions hidden beneath the original thought. Here is an example:

You wake up in pain and think, "I'm so useless." First you ask yourself, "If this is true, why does it upset me?" "So what?" or "What's the worst that could happen?"

↓

You write, "I can never do anything anybody wants me to do." Ask yourself again, "If this is true, why does it upset me?" "So what?" "What's the worst that could happen?"

↓

"Now my friend will hate me because I'm unreliable." Ask yourself, "So what?"

↓

"Soon I'll have no friends." Ask yourself, "So what?"

↓

"I'm afraid of being alone." Ask yourself, "So what?"

↓

"Being alone is the worst thing that can happen to me."

And so on. In the example above, the underlying fear of being alone can make any situation that isolates you the source of depression and panic. Once you know where the panic is coming from, you can take steps to cope with the loneliness.

At the end of this chapter is a questionnaire called the Dysfunctional Attitude Scale (DAS) (an unfortunate name but helpful tool). Completing it can help you identify the troubling assumptions that you harbor, often unknowingly. These distortions make you vulnerable to daily stresses. My colleagues and I have found the DAS very helpful.

Following the questionnaire is an explanation of how to interpret your answers. For example, if your DAS score is lowest in Perfectionism and Achievement, you are likely to believe that you must achieve perfectly all the time. Your self-talk probably sounds like this: "If I can't work, I don't deserve to do anything fun"; "If I make a mistake, I'm stupid and inadequate"; "I'm a terrible father if I can't play baseball with my kids." Challenging such thoughts is part of getting to drive your own yellow school bus—or, to borrow another metaphor, get rid of those old tapes and make your own.

The Narrative Repair

"The narrative repair" is the technique of writing about stressful or traumatic events. Keeping diaries or journals is certainly not new, but research into the powerful healing effects of putting words down on paper is. James Pennebaker describes his own research in his book *Opening Up: The Healing Power of Expressing Emotions* (see "Supplementary Reading"). Other studies also show that writing about your stresses and traumas can be therapeutic. As people continue to write, they can make sense of what has happened to them. This is the narrative repair. Bringing meaning to the pain experience can be an important step in healing and in decreasing long-term disability. This kind of writing is not a form of complaining or a substitute for acting on a problem. It can allow you to identify a starting point for addressing frustrations or beginning to problem solve. Writing that is self-reflective (not self-absorbed or intellectual) will be the most therapeutic.

Changing Self-Talk Practice

The techniques I've been describing will not make you stressless. However, they can help you to control your responses to life's minor and major hassles. You will feel differently when you can describe what is going on and determine your options. David Burns's books are highly recommended for further work in this area (see "Supplementary Reading").

Try practicing with all three of the techniques presented here. Changing how you feel by changing what you say to yourself may be an unusual idea for you. You may need practice to become skilled at it. In the beginning, you may only be able to identify your thoughts after the fact. Eventually, however, you will be able to start questioning as soon as you start hearing your inner chatter. You will know when you have captured the thoughts that created your negative emotions, because just by reading them you will re-create the emotions. But beware of the "Why me?" questions. Go beyond them to the assumptions or expectations that underlie such questions. You will know when you've hit upon an adequate way to change a thought, because you will feel better and more in control.

Now let's take a look at what happened to Joan (see the quote at the beginning of the chapter). By the end of the program, her thinking had undergone a transformation. The following is the beginning of a poem she wrote, based on a dream she had during the program:

> A friend showed me a grey cement urn, the size of a well. It opened slightly.
> Inside were limbs, arms and legs floating in a thin, dark liquid.
> A man dove to the bottom and brought my body to the surface. It was
>   not dead, only half dead—kept alive somehow by a mask and snorkel.
> I was afraid to look at it, but I did—
> When I saw that it was me, I turned to my friend and husband and said
>   with utter joy: "I'm so glad to be living."
> I watched the man lift my body from the urn and begin to walk with it.
>   My body slowly began to come to life.
> The man led my body onto a boat where a crowd was gathered to watch.
>   The two walked through the middle of the crowd of people.
> As they did so, my body was transformed. It became filled with light and
>   covered by white flowing garments. The head became covered with
>   long, golden hair.
> At the bow of the boat, my body sailed off into the sky and the crowd of
>   people cheered.
> I thought to myself as I watched: "I am beautiful."

The Role of Psychology in Chronic Pain

There has been a great deal of debate in medicine about whether or not chronic pain is simply a physical sign of psychological trauma, depression, or hysteria. Many believe that chronic pain has a psychological or psychosomatic cause. These psychological theories have gained popularity in part because of medicine's separation of mind and body. In addition, ignorance about chronic pain contributes to the idea that what can't be seen must be "psychological."

Many doctors emphasize either the body or the mind in their therapies. A body doctor rarely explores the emotional or psychological signs of living in pain, and a mind doctor seldom if ever physically examines a patient. Yet, when I listen to chronic pain patients describe their physical, emotional, and social limitations, it is very clear to me that mind *and* body are intimately involved in the experience of chronic pain. It is important to make psychological diagnoses so that appropriate treatment can be prescribed; however, there may be too much psychological labeling of chronic pain patients who do not get better. This only increases everyone's frustration and devalues patients' experience; it does not clarify how best to treat them. Let's explore some of the psychological labels that are commonly used in chronic pain.

Common Psychological Labels in Chronic Pain

Depression

In the absence of pain, feeling sad or worthless and having trouble sleeping or eating may be symptoms of depression. But in a person experiencing pain, these common symptoms can be a sign of the struggle to live with the pain, which can be quite disruptive. The treatment of a person with chronic pain may include antidepressants, but they should be part of a comprehensive treatment plan.

Depressed patients also complain of bodily aches and pains; their pain complaints usually go away when the depression is successfully treated. In chronic pain, the sensation doesn't go away with the treatment of the depression, although the pain *experience* may improve.

Hysteria

Many women patients with chronic pain are incorrectly labeled as "hysterical," simply because they are female and complain about unexplained pain. "Hysteria" is a term with great historical interest. In medical writings as recently as the last century, the womb (in Greek, *hystera*) was considered to be the source of many female problems. It supposedly made a woman prone to moodiness, fickleness, irritability, and multiple physical complaints. These "abnormal," "hysterical" behaviors contrasted with the supposed calm, steady, rational behavior of the "normal" (that is, male) population.

Hysteria as a mental illness was described as early as the 16th century. Again, it was described as occurring primarily in women (though men were occasionally described as experiencing the illness as well). Sigmund Freud influenced the current psychiatric understanding of hysteria. He wrote extensively about the cause and treatment of this mysterious loss of physical function. It could involve almost any part of the body and was associated with psychological traumas (usually involving sexual conflict). The hysterical patients were also characterized by a particular emotional response called *la belle indifférence*. That is, they did not seem to care about their loss of function, such as their inability to speak or walk. Typically, patients with chronic pain care very much about their loss of function.

Use of the term "hysterical" to describe a frightened female (or male) patient with chronic pain does not appear to be appropriate or accurate, even if the response seems exaggerated. The fact that X-ray or laboratory findings cannot identify the cause of chronic pain does not justify a diagnosis of hysteria or the label of "hysterical." We would do better to observe that pain behaviors are signs of suffering that occur in a woman *or* man with chronic pain. We also need to realize that "appropriate behaviors" are culturally and socially determined and as such are subject to interpretation and bias.

Hypochondriasis

Some people are intensely preoccupied with and worried about their health. They are sensitive to the physical sensations of normal body functioning and may become alarmed by things like their own normal heartbeat. They are rarely reassured by their doctors' examinations or tests. Such people are referred to as hypochondriacs.

It is easy to see how the label of "hypochondriac" might be misapplied to chronic pain patients. For example, in fibromyalgia (see Appendix A), the pain is ill defined, diffuse, intermittent, and migratory; there is no specific laboratory test that can confirm the diagnosis. In such cases, it is essential that a careful history and examination be performed. The pattern of symptoms, the presence of tender points, and the absence of positive results for rheumatoid arthritis or lupus on laboratory tests can help make the diagnosis of fibromyalgia. In addition, the willingness of patients with fibromyalgia to be active participants in their pain management, working in partnership with their health care providers, demonstrates a healthy coping response. This would be an unlikely response in patients suffering from hypochondriasis.

Malingering

There appears to be considerable paranoia on the part of many insurance companies and physicians about chronic pain sufferers being "malingerers"—people who only pretend to be ill. Such paranoia generates blame and distrust between health care providers and patients. This state of affairs is probably due in part to the "who's to blame," litigious atmosphere in which medicine is currently practiced. It's hard enough for physicians and other care providers to make accurate diagnoses and treat symptoms, without also wondering whether the symptoms being reported are "real." The lack of clearly defined explanations for chronic pain also confuses practitioners about the reality of the pain. Further misunderstanding is created when physicians perceive that a patient has somehow failed at or sabotaged "usually successful" therapy and when patients perceive that the physician has failed to deliver pain relief.

If a health care provider and a patient in pain are to have a successful therapeutic relationship, blame and distrust must be put aside. Chronic pain is not a failure on either the patient's or the physician's part. Chronic pain is real, not imaginary or invented. For many patients, it's not a curable problem, but the symptoms can be reduced.

A patient's search for the meaning of the pain can lead him or her to focus on finding someone to blame, particularly when pain occurs after an accident. Although the prospect of being compensated through a legal action or worker's compensation may influence the experience of pain, it does not appear to create pain in the majority of individuals. As discussed in Chapter 6, many a compensation scenario is associated with anger and frustration, which can interfere with healing and can worsen the pain experience. When the legal system, worker's compensation, or a disability insurer becomes involved in an individual's case, there is often a lengthening of the normal grieving process and a delay in coming to acceptance of the chronic pain condition. This delay is not malingering, however.

In short, patients are responsible for clearly and accurately reporting their pain experience, physicians are responsible for thorough evaluation and treatment, and external systems need to provide compensation in a timely and just manner.

Posttraumatic Stress Disorder

Considerable attention is currently being given to posttraumatic stress disorder (PTSD). Some theorists believe that certain types of chronic pain (for example, headaches, abdominal pain, and pelvic pain) are really the psychological signs of sexual or physical abuse that occurred years before.

Another explanation, however, may be that for those with chronic pain *and* significant physical or emotional trauma, chronic pain *feels* like being abused again. Both patients in pain and people with PTSD feel anxiety, vulnerability, and lack of control, and they may not be believed. The PTSD may not cause the pain in these circumstances, but it may compound the experience of physical pain because of the similar qualities of these two emotion-laden experiences. The psychological distress of PTSD needs treating, and so does the physical pain. The desire to reduce the emotional pain of trauma as well as the physical pain makes the use of opioids a particular challenge. It is extremely important in these situations that patients receive a comprehensive approach to treatment that addresses mind, body, and spirit.

Before multiple surgical or medical procedures are performed, it is important to explore whether PTSD is also present. For example, in persistent pelvic pain, the pain may not reach a level where surgery is considered if the coexisting factor of PTSD is treated as well. The relationship between PTSD and pain is an important connection to be explored, because the healing must take place at multiple levels— in the memories of the mind *and* the body.

Summary

- We know that certain ways of thinking are commonly associated with disability in chronic pain, for example, catastrophizing, denial, avoidance, and wishful thinking.

- Automatic thoughts or self-talk can affect the way you feel. If you can change your negative self-talk, you can actually change how you feel.

- Our cultural beliefs and vocabulary influence how we perceive the world around us, our predisposition for short-term planning leaves us vulnerable to long-term consequences, and gender, as well as culture, influences our interpersonal communication.

- Albert Ellis developed rational–emotive therapy to challenge irrational beliefs and replace them with more realistic ones.

- David Burns identified 10 types of cognitive distortions that can lead to negative emotions.

- Monitor your self-talk and physical/emotional responses to stressful situations. This helps you to evaluate and begin to change these responses. Carefully examine anger and thoughts of "Why me?"

- Changing thoughts associated with negative emotional states allows you to identify your options and gain greater control over your responses to life's difficulties. Three techniques are presented:

  —Challenging the reality of your self-talk

  —Clarifying the problem and developing an action plan

  —The vertical arrow ("So what?") technique for those more difficult-to-reach agendas

- Psychological labels for chronic pain patients may be helpful when used to understand the process and formulate a treatment plan.

Exploration Tasks

1. Using the "Daily Record of Automatic Thoughts (Self-Talk)": Keep track of what you are thinking whenever you experience a negative emotional state (sadness, anxiety, fear, or jealousy) or whenever you are feeling increased physical tension or pain. (You have automatic thoughts with positive emotional states, too, but clearly you don't need to work on changing those emotional states.) Copy and use the "Daily Record of Automatic Thoughts (Self-Talk)" provided at the end of this book.

   - First identify and record the event or situation associated with negative (sad, self-defeated, anxious) emotions. For example: *Pain flare-up.*

   - Write down your thoughts (capturing them on paper): *"I can't take it anymore."*

Sample Daily Record of Automatic Thoughts (Self-Talk)

Date	Situation	Automatic thoughts	Physical response	Emotional response	Cognitive distortion	Changed thought
Example: 1/02/08	Pain flare-up	Can't take this. I can't do anything.	↑ tension crying	Helpless Frustrated	All or nothing Magnification	1. Pain increases are scary. 2. I've been through this before. 3. I have tools I can apply to get through this. 4. This is what I'll do . . .

Adapted from Aaron T. Beck et al., *Cognitive Therapy of Depression* (New York: Guilford Press, 1979). Copyright 1979 by Aaron T. Beck, A. John Rush, Brian F. Shaw, and Gary Emery. Adapted by permission.

- Write down the physical symptoms you experience at these stressful times: *"Muscle tension, heartburn."*

- Write down the emotional response: *"Out of control, helpless."*

- Write down the distortion, the belief behind the thoughts: *"If I can't take it maybe someone else will [wishful thinking]. It's beyond my control and there is nothing I can do to help myself [all-or-nothing thinking, catastrophic thinking]."*

- Using one of the three techniques, see if you can challenge unrealistic thoughts and distortions. Come up with more realistic, action-oriented thoughts and phrases: *"The reality is that I can take it and have. I don't have to like it. I have many things I can do to manage my pain flare-up."*

2. Certain techniques can help you identify, capture, and change your self-talk.

   A. The regular practice of RR techniques (see Chapter 3) encourages self-observation. If you have not been practicing a daily RR technique, you may have more trouble capturing these quick thoughts. Consider increasing your commitment to daily RR practice.

   B. Journaling can help you identify the automatic thoughts that you may have trouble observing, identifying, or admitting. The most common problem when people begin to start monitoring their self-talk is that they do not go beyond describing their mood. They do not explore the thoughts that are responsible for the mood. They go immediately to problem solving. Although problem solving is where we want to go with these exercises, you may not be ready yet. Unless you want always to be a victim, you first need to see what drives these ever-present self-defeating thoughts. That means identifying the thoughts that make you sad, angry, or anxious and the beliefs that are driving them—fear of losing control, of not being loved, of being used by others, and so forth. Journaling is a way of taking the time to capture the thoughts, all of them, and exploring the assumptions behind them. Usually people find they have a few common distortions that run through most of their self-talk. Taking the time to reflect on these common scenarios will allow you to gain more mastery over them. Write about a stressful event for 10–20 minutes, letting whatever comes up flow out onto the paper (or if this is difficult because of your particular site of pain, use a tape recorder). You do not have to share it with anyone. See what comes up. What are the familiar themes? Phrases? Do not be surprised if you feel the emotion more intensely. You are getting to the roots of your despair. Only after you get it all out on paper can you start working on changing the self-statements, challenging the reality of what you have said and identifying the distortions. If anger is a dominant theme, try the next exercise.

3. Anger, as I pointed out before, is a challenge. There are many reasons people become angry; this exercise deals with only a few of them. People injured by someone else in an accident or at work often feel angry at the other person. They may feel vulnerable and uncertain about whether they can ever feel safe again. This can be quite distressful. Being a victim feels awful. But why? Can you capture or identify why you feel angry? (Substituting the word "hurt" or "frustration" for "anger" may make this easier for some people.) For example: *"I feel angry (hurt, frustrated) because that person was careless when he ran the red light and could have killed me!"*

I feel (   ) because . . . _____

_____

_____

Can you identify how the other person may see things from *his or her* point of view? *"It was a mistake, I didn't mean to, I shouldn't have been talking on the cell phone, it was stupid."*

_____

_____

When you think about the threatening incident, what does your body do in response to the angry thoughts? (*breath holding, increased muscle tension, increased blood pressure*)

_____

_____

_____

When you think about the incident from the other person's viewpoint, how does your body respond?

_____

_____

_____

What are the advantages to staying angry? What might be the disadvantages?

_____

_____

_____

Can you identify ways to suffer less physically because of your anger? (*relaxation techniques, breathing through the tension while thinking of your anger*)

_____

_____

_____

Can you identify ways to suffer less emotionally from your anger? (*consider meditation; look to the future for what I can do, not to the past for what I've lost*)

_____

_____

_____

4. Complete the Dysfunctional Attitude Scale (DAS) provided at the end of this chapter. After you identify the categories in which you scored the lowest (the minus numbers or the lowest positive numbers), look at the five questions composing each category and identify the irrational beliefs or cognitive distortions associated with them. Use this information to help challenge some of the irrational self-talk you engage in from time to time and to identify patterns in various situations that disrupt your peace of mind. You may feel upset by what you find out, but remember that the truth can set you free!

5. Making use of the Dysfunctional Attitude Scale

When you find yourself reacting to your pain or life events in a negative way with frustration, feelings of defeat, giving up, giving in . . .

A. STOP, TAKE A DEEP BREATH.

B. Ask yourself, "What is going on here? Are these my old tapes or assumptions playing out here?"

C. "Where do I have control here? What can I do?"

D. PRACTICE, PRACTICE, PRACTICE.

6. Write out a goal that you want to accomplish related to this chapter. As always, make sure your goal is a behavioral task that you can measure in terms of the steps *you* will take to accomplish it. Here is an example:

Goal: *Keep track of my automatic thoughts when I become aware that I am de-pressed or anxious.*

Steps to take to reach that goal:

A. *Copy the chart at the back of the book and carry it in my pocket.*

B. *If I can't capture the automatic thoughts, I'll use the writing exercise to write about each incident and see what comes up.*

C. *After completing the DAS, I will examine the nature of the situations that were associated with the depression or anxiety and see if they match any of my self-defeating attitudes identified by the DAS.*

Now it's your turn.

Goal: _____

Steps to take to reach that goal:

A. _____

B. _____

C. _____

D. _____

In addition, list contingency plans. That is, identify what obstacles might get in the way of your accomplishing this goal. What solutions can you devise to work toward insuring the success of this goal?

	Obstacles	**Solutions**
A.	_____	_____
B.	_____	_____
C.	_____	_____
D.	_____	_____

Supplementary Reading

The following books provide additional ideas and observations regarding how and why we think the way we do:

Arthur J. Barsky and Emily C. Deans, *Feeling Better: A 6-Week Mind–Body Program to Ease Your Chronic Symptoms* (New York: HarperCollins, 2006).
David Burns, *The Feeling Good Handbook* (New York: Plume, 1999).

David Burns, *Ten Days to Self-Esteem* (New York: Quill/William Morrow, 1999).

Robert Cialdini, *Influence: The Psychology of Persuasion* (New York: Collins, 2006).

Albert Ellis, *How to Make Yourself Happy and Remarkably Less Disturbable* (Manassas Park, VA: Impact, 1999).

W. Doyle Gentry, *Anger Management for Dummies* (Hoboken, NJ: Wiley, 2007).

Edward T. Hall, *Beyond Culture* (New York: Anchor, 1977).

Thich Nhat Hanh, *Anger: Wisdom for Cooling the Flames* (NewYork: Riverhead Books, 2001).

Matthew McKay and Peter Rogers, *The Anger Control Workbook* (Oakland, CA: New Harbinger Publications, 2000).

Robert Ornstein, *Evolution of Consciousness* (New York: Touchstone, 1992).

Robert Ornstein, *The Psychology of Consciousness, Second Edition* (New York: Penguin Books, 1996).

James Pennebaker, *Opening Up: The Healing Power of Expressing Emotions* (New York: Guilford Press, 1997).

Martin Seligman, *Learned Optimism* (New York: Pocket Books, 1998).

Idries Shah, *The Pleasantries of the Incredible Mulla Nasrudin* (London: Octagon Press, 1983).

Idries Shah, *Reflections* (London: Octagon Press, 1983).

Idries Shah, *The Subtleties of the Inimitable Mulla Nasrudin* and *The Exploits of the Incomparable Mulla Nasrudin* (London: Octagon Press, 1989).

Deborah Tannen, *You Just Don't Understand: Women and Men in Conversation* (New York: Ballantine Books, 1991).

Beverly Thorn, *Cognitive Therapy for Chronic Pain: A Step-by-Step Guide* (New York: Guilford Press, 2004).

Hendria Weisinger, *Dr. Weisinger's Anger Workout Book* (New York: Quill, 1985).

Denise Winn, *The Manipulated Mind: Brainwashing, Conditioning and Manipulation* (Los Altos, CA: Malor Books, 2000).

Dysfunctional Attitude Scale (DAS)

Instructions

As you fill out the questionnaire, indicate how much you agree or disagree with each attitude. When you are finished, an answer key will let you score your answers and generate a profile of your personal values systems. This will show your areas of psychological strength and vulnerability.

Answering the test is quite simple. After each of the 35 attitudes, put a check in the column that represents your estimate of how you think *most* of the time. Be sure to choose only one answer for each attitude. Because we are all different, there is no "right" or "wrong" answer to any statement. To decide whether a given attitude is typical of your own philosophy, recall how you look at things most of the time.

Statement	Agree strongly	Agree slightly	Neutral	Disagree slightly	Disagree very much
1. Criticism will obviously upset the person who receives the criticism.	____	____	____	____	____
2. It is best to give up my own interests in order to please other people.	____	____	____	____	____
3. I need other people's approval in order to be happy.	____	____	____	____	____
4. If someone important to me expects me to do something, then I really should do it.	____	____	____	____	____
5. My value as a person depends greatly on what others think of me.	____	____	____	____	____
6. I cannot find happiness without being loved by another person.	____	____	____	____	____
7. If others dislike you, you are bound to be less happy.	____	____	____	____	____
8. If people whom I care about reject me, it means there is something wrong with me.	____	____	____	____	____

(cont.)

Dysfunctional Attitude Scale *(cont.)*

Statement	Agree strongly	Agree slightly	Neutral	Disagree slightly	Disagree very much
9. If a person I love does not love me, it means I am unlovable.	____	____	____	____	____
10. Being isolated from others is bound to lead to unhappiness.	____	____	____	____	____
11. If I am to be a worthwhile person, I must be truly outstanding in at least one major respect.	____	____	____	____	____
12. I must be a useful, productive, creative person or life has no purpose.	____	____	____	____	____
13. People who have good ideas are more worthy than those who do not.	____	____	____	____	____
14. If I do not do as well as other people, it means I am inferior.	____	____	____	____	____
15. If I fail at my work, then I am a failure as a person.	____	____	____	____	____
16. If you cannot do something well, there is little point in doing it at all.	____	____	____	____	____
17. It is shameful for a person to display his or her weaknesses.	____	____	____	____	____
18. A person should try to be the best at everything he or she undertakes.	____	____	____	____	____
19. I should be upset if I make a mistake.	____	____	____	____	____
20. If I don't set the highest standards for myself, I am likely to end up a second-rate person.	____	____	____	____	____
21. If I strongly believe I deserve something, I have reason to expect I should get it.	____	____	____	____	____
22. It is necessary to become frustrated if you find obstacles to getting what you want.	____	____	____	____	____
23. If I put other people's needs before my own, they should help me when I need something from them.	____	____	____	____	____

Statement	Agree strongly	Agree slightly	Neutral	Disagree slightly	Disagree very much
24. If I am a good husband or wife, then my spouse is bound to love me.	____	____	____	____	____
25. If I do nice things for someone, I can anticipate that he or she will respect and treat me just as well as I treat them.	____	____	____	____	____
26. I should assume responsibility for how people feel and behave if they are close to me.	____	____	____	____	____
27. If I criticize the way someone does something and he or she becomes angry or depressed, this means I have upset him or her.	____	____	____	____	____
28. To be a good, worthwhile, moral person, I must try to help everyone who needs it.	____	____	____	____	____
29. If a child is having emotional or behavioral difficulties, this shows that the child's parents have failed in some important respect.	____	____	____	____	____
30. I should be able to please everybody.	____	____	____	____	____
31. I cannot expect to control how I feel when something bad happens.	____	____	____	____	____
32. There is no point in trying to change upsetting emotions because they are a valid and inevitable part of daily living.	____	____	____	____	____
33. My moods are primarily created by factors that are largely beyond my control, such as the past, body chemistry, hormone cycles, biorhythms, chance, or fate.	____	____	____	____	____
34. My happiness is largely dependent on what happens to me.	____	____	____	____	____
35. People who have the marks of success (good looks, social status, wealth, or fame) are bound to be happier than those who do not.	____	____	____	____	____

Adapted from David Burns, *Feeling Good: The New Mood Therapy* (New York: William Morrow, 1980). Copyright 1980 by David Burns, MD. Adapted by permission of the author and the publisher.

Scoring the DAS

Now that you have completed the DAS, you can score it in the following way. Score your answer to each of the thirty-five attitudes according to this key:

Agree strongly	Agree slightly	Neutral	Disagree slightly	Disagree very much
–2	–1	0	+1	+2

Now add up your score on the first five attitudes. These measure your tendency to measure your worth in term of the opinions of others and the amount of approval or criticism you receive. Suppose your scores on these five items were +2, +1, –1, +2, 0. Then your total score for these five questions would be +4.

Proceed in this way to add up your score for items 1 through 5, 6 through 10, 11 through 15, 16 through 20, 21 through 25, 26 through 30, and 31 through 35, and record these as illustrated in the following example:

Scoring example:

Value system	Attitudes	Individual scores	Total score
I. Approval	1 through 5	+2, +1, –1, +2, 0	+4
II. Love	6 through 10	–2, –1, –2, –2, 0	–7
III. Achievement	11 through 15	+1, +1, 0, 0, –2	0
IV. Perfectionism	16 through 20	+2, +2, +1, +1, +1	+7
V. Entitlement	21 through 25	+1, +1, –1, +1, 0	+2
VI. Omnipotence	26 through 30	–2, –1, 0, –1, +1	–3
VII. Autonomy	31 through 35	–2, –2, –1, –2, –2	–9

Record your actual scores here:

Value system	Attitudes	Individual scores	Total score
I. Approval	1 through 5	_____	_____
II. Love	6 through 10	_____	_____
III. Achievement	11 through 15	_____	_____
IV. Perfectionism	16 through 20	_____	_____
V. Entitlement	21 through 25	_____	_____
VI. Omnipotence	26 through 30	_____	_____
VII. Autonomy	31 through 35	_____	_____

(cont.)

Each cluster of five items from the scale measures one of seven value systems. Your total score for each cluster of five items can range from +10 to −10. Now you can read about each variable and develop your personal philosophy profile.

Interpreting Your DAS Score

I. *Approval* (items 1–5): These items assess your tendency to base your self-esteem on others' reactions to you. A positive score (between 0 and +10) indicates that you are independent with a healthy sense of your own worth, even when confronted with criticism and disapproval. A negative score (between 0 and −10) indicates that you are very dependent, because you evaluate yourself through other people's eyes. You are vulnerable to anxiety and depression when others criticize you or are angry with you.

II. *Love* (items 6–10): These items assess your tendency to base your self-worth on whether or not you are loved. A positive score (between 0 and +10) indicates that you see love as desirable but that you have a wide range of other interests that you also find fulfilling and gratifying. Hence, love is not a requirement for your happiness or self-esteem. A negative score (between 0 and −10) indicates that you see love as a "need" without which you cannot survive or be happy. You tend to adopt inferior roles in relationships with people you care about for fear of alienating them. You may even resort to manipulative behavior in order to get people's affection and attention. Ironically, this needy, greedy attitude often drives people away, thus intensifying your loneliness.

III. *Achievement* (items 11–15): These items assess your tendency to base your self-esteem on whether or not you are productive. A positive score (between 0 and +10) indicates that you enjoy creativity and productivity but do not see them as a necessary road to self-esteem and satisfaction. A negative score (between 0 and −10) indicates that you are a workaholic. Your sense of self-worth and your capacity for joy are dependent on your productivity. If your business slumps, if you retire, or if you become ill or inactive, you will be at risk for an emotional crash.

IV. *Perfectionism* (items 16–20): These items assess your tendency to base your self-worth on your ability to avoid failures and mistakes. A positive score (between 0 and +10) indicates that you have the capacity to set meaningful, flexible, and appropriate standards. You enjoy processes and experiences for their own sake, and are not exclusively fixated on outcomes. You don't have to be outstanding at everything. You don't fear mistakes but see them as opportunities to grow and learn. A negative score (between 0 and −10) indicates that you demand perfection in yourself—mistakes are taboo, failure is "worse than death," and even negative emotions are a disaster. You are living with impossible and unrealistic personal standards, and life becomes a joyless, tedious treadmill.

V. *Entitlement* (items 21–25): These items measure the extent to which you feel you deserve the best out of life, simply because you're you. A positive score (between 0 and +10) indicates that you don't always feel automatically entitled to things, so you negotiate for what you want and often get it. You realize there is no inherent reason why things should always go your way. You experience a negative outcome as a disappointment, not a tragedy, knowing that you can't expect "justice" at all times. You are patient and persistent, with high frustration tolerance. A negative score (between 0 and −10) indicates that you feel entitled to things (success, love, happiness, etc.). You expect and demand that your wants be met by other people and the universe in general because of your inherent goodness and hard work. When this does not happen, you feel depressed and inadequate; you may become irate. Thus you expend much energy being frustrated, sad, and/or mad.

VI. *Omnipotence* (items 26–30): These items measure your tendency to see yourself as the center of your personal universe and to hold yourself responsible for much of what goes on around you. A positive score (between 0 and +10) indicates that you know the joy that comes from accepting that you are not the center of the universe. Since you are not in control of other adults, you are not ultimately responsible for them, but only for yourself. You relate to others as a collaborator. You aren't threatened when others disagree with your ideas or fail to follow your advice. People frequently listen to you and respect your ideas, because you do not polarize them with insistence that they must agree with you. Your relationships with people are characterized by mutuality instead of dependency. A negative score (between 0 and –10) indicates that you blame others who are not really under your control. Consequently, you are plagued by guilt and self-condemnation. The attitude that you should be omnipotent and all-powerful leaves you anxious and ineffective.

VII. *Autonomy* (items 31–35): These items measure your ability to find happiness within yourself. A positive score (between 0 and +10) indicates that all your moods are a result of your thoughts and attitudes. You assume responsibility for your feelings because you recognize that they are ultimately created by you. A negative score (between 0 and –10) indicates that you are trapped in the belief that your potential for joy and self-esteem comes from the outside. Your moods are the victim of external factors. This puts you at a disadvantage, because everything is ultimately beyond your control.

Adapted from David Burns, *Feeling Good: The New Mood Therapy* (New York: William Morrow, 1980). Copyright 1980 by David Burns, MD. Adapted by permission of the author and the publisher.

A Final Word on the DAS

The DAS is not an infallible test, and you may not agree with the results. If so, you're not alone; this questionnaire has been met with some of the strongest comments in our pain program. However, the overwhelming majority of people find the scale to be very valuable in identifying self-defeating attitudes, once their objections or their self-critical thoughts about the results ("I must really be crazy," "I didn't realize I was so dysfunctional") are put aside. It is amazing how accurately it identifies and predicts the types of scenarios that push people's vulnerable buttons. Give it a try.

6

Adopting Healthy Attitudes

There was once an old farmer who had a mare. One day the mare broke through a fence and ran away. "Now you have no horse to pull your plow at planting time," the neighbors said. "What bad luck this is."

"Good luck, bad luck," replied the farmer. "Who knows?"

The next week the mare returned, bringing with her two wild stallions. "With three horses you are now a rich man," the neighbors said. "What good fortune this is."

"Good fortune, bad fortune," replied the farmer. "Who knows?"

That afternoon the farmer's only son tried to tame one of the stallions, but he was thrown and broke a leg. "Now you have no one to help you with planting," the neighbors said. "What bad luck this is."

"Good luck, bad luck," replied the farmer. "Who knows?"

The next day the emperor's soldiers rode into town and conscripted the oldest son of every family, but the farmer's son was left behind because of his broken leg. "Your son is the only eldest in the province who has not been taken from his family," the neighbors said. "What good fortune this is . . ."

—*A Zen story about an old Chinese farmer (retold in* The Wellness Book, *p. 460; see Chapter 2, "Supplementary Reading")*

This Zen story illustrates a flexible attitude. In essence, it demonstrates that whatever people's interpretations of events may be, there is always considerable uncertainty in life. Developing an ease with uncertainty is a way of adapting to life's daily hassles and stresses. For people like you, who now find themselves living in pain, this adaptability can be crucial for coping. Medical and scientific research by Seligman (2006), Fawzy et al. (1993), Nelson et al. (2000), and Williams and Williams (1998) has found that there are numerous health benefits for those who can shed rigid, destructive lifestyles, behaviors, and attitudes and adopt more flexible, positive ones. These benefits include decreased risk factors for heart disease, reduced recurrences of heart attacks, improved immune system function, and increased life span for cancer patients. Indeed, we are only just beginning to understand and appreciate the power of adaptability and positive attitudes.

The term "attitude" is used here to mean a psychological characteristic that a person usually adopts without thinking about it. Attitudes are the result of many influences, such as culture, family, learning, and perhaps genetics. We all have attitudes; they help us make daily decisions without weighing every single one of them. Attitudes can become a problem when they are negative and inflexible and make it harder for us to adapt to changing circumstances.

For example, if your attitude is that you can't control what happens to you, then you may not see the point of behaving in healthier ways. You may say, "If I'm going to be in pain, why should I bother to stop smoking or follow a low-fat diet?" To take another example, you're in pain but think you must do your housekeeping the same way you did it before the pain. Chances are that you will suffer more and still not have a clean house. When you find yourself with attitudes like these, you need to stop and take a look at them.

Learned helplessness and anger/hostility are common problematic attitudes among the chronic pain patients I see. I discuss these particular attitudes next because they interfere to the greatest extent with effective coping and problem solving. By contrast, attitudes such as stress hardiness, optimism, empathy, and altruism can help ease the uncertainty of life in general and life with chronic pain in particular.

Problematic Attitudes

Learned Helplessness

If you put a rat in a cage and give the rat an electric shock every time it presses a bar, then the rat will soon learn to stop pressing the bar. But if you randomly give a rat electric shocks that it cannot control, it will begin to act anxious and hypervigilant. After some time, if this rat is put through a maze, it will not be able to learn as it did before. It will become withdrawn and may stop eating. If this goes on long enough, it will make no effort to help itself even if it's given a chance and even if the shocks have stopped. This behavior is called "learned helplessness." The rat has thoroughly learned that there is nothing it can do to change its unpleasant circumstances. This attitude then affects how it approaches even the things over which it does have control.

Many patients experiencing chronic pain adopt an attitude of learned helplessness. They may ask, or even beg, for help but find it difficult to believe that anything they do for themselves will help their pain. This attitude, however, is a self-fulfilling prophecy. It means that they stay helpless and that nothing changes. Practicing the skills discussed in this book, and doing the exploration tasks and other exercises, will help you find those places where you do have control. You can learn new ways of living with pain.

Anger/Hostility

Anger and Responsibility

Chapter 5 mentions that working with feelings of anger requires a slightly different approach than just identifying or changing self-talk. Some people hold on to anger and hostility; if this is you, you need to explore why. Anger and hostility often involve blaming someone or something else. The blamed party is held responsible for the angry feelings. The need to hold someone or something responsible for suffering can be very strong. Moreover, there are times when anger is both appropriate and justified. It can be a basis for constructive action. But simply holding on to anger or hostility can be destructive to the victim. Many studies show this: for example, it can raise the risk of cardiovascular disease (see Williams and Williams in "Supplementary Reading"). Blaming others for one's misery only gives away the control you could have. The pent-up anger spreads ever wider, causing depression, anxiety, self-doubt, and more anger.

Some people protest that accepting responsibility for the way they feel is the same as admitting that they have done something wrong or giving in; this is not the case. Many angry patients fear that if they let go of their anger there will be nothing left of them. The anger has become a self-sustaining force in their lives. Again, too, depression and anxiety often underlie the anger or are even created by it. Staying angry may help these patients to avoid facing such feelings. Who suffers by hanging on to such negative emotions? When she realized the self-destructive nature of her anger one patient said, "I've been letting someone else live rent-free in my head!"

As noted in Chapter 5, patients whose pain is the result of injury from an accident at work or from someone else's negligence are understandably very angry at times. However, many patients involved in worker's compensation claims, litigation, or the like find themselves fighting against a mighty and invisible adversary. Their feelings of being wronged and misunderstood, their attempts to find an explanation or compensation for the suffering, feed the "me against them" attitude. One of my patients was suing someone because she had slipped on the ice in that person's driveway and injured her back. I asked her, "Who would you blame if you slipped on the ice in your own driveway?" She replied without a pause, "Me, I guess."

Coping with anger involves recognizing your own responsibilities, including the responsibility to identify your automatic thoughts. For example, you may be thinking something like this: "Someone must pay for my suffering. The accident that injured me was an unforgivable event, and I will not be comforted until the wrong has been corrected." Once these thoughts have been divulged, it is necessary to identify where your responsibility ends and that of others begins. Forgiveness may be described as coming to accept the injustices that you have experienced. It is a difficult and arduous process. However, it can help you clarify who's responsible for what after an injury.

The Five Phases of Forgiveness

Beverly Flanigan, a psychologist who has studied the process of forgiveness, describes five phases leading to forgiveness in her book *Forgiving the Unforgivable: Overcoming the Bitter Legacy of Intimate Wounds* (see "Supplementary Reading"). The book is about forgiving betrayal in personal relationships, but you can apply the process to forgiving physical injuries as well.

Phase 1: Naming the Injury. The first phase gives you as the injured person the opportunity to clarify what the wrongful act was and to explore how you interpret the significance or meaning of that act.

For example, say the car you were driving was hit from behind and you received a neck injury. Perhaps the wrongful act committed by the other driver was not leaving enough space between cars, or speeding, or not paying attention to slowing traffic. When you explore the significance of the wrongful act, you may find that you take it as a personal violation. Furthermore, if the other person has never apologized, you may feel further justified in seeking punishment for the person's wrongdoing. However, the implicit moral rule "Thou shalt do no harm" may complicate your feelings about this act.

If lawyers become involved, this important phase may be delayed until the case comes to court, many months or years later. If you don't name the injury and explore its significance for you, you may also not be able to begin to admit that the painful consequences are permanent and take the steps necessary to cope (Phase 2). In addition, the possibility of talking to the injurer will be limited to depositions. You will be kept from identifying with any human weakness on his or her part (such as having made a mistake). Clearly, being wronged is painful; when the effects are physical and long term, there is a wish to be compensated at many levels. This is appropriate, but if the phases of forgiveness are arrested at the beginning, there may only be the external resolution (the settlement) without an internal resolution of the distress.

Phase 2: Claiming the Injury. Phase 2 of the process involves admitting that the injury is permanent and that the pain is yours to cope with. You stop blaming your suffering on the injurer, and you stop denying that you have the responsibility and the need to go forward.

Phase 3: Blaming the Injurer. In Phase 3, someone is held accountable for causing the harm. In a situation involving a motor vehicle accident, such as the example given above, it is usually the other driver. Other situations involving injury may not be so clear-cut. If you have experienced a work-related injury, it may be the nature of the job—for example, the repetitive motion involved in typing on a keyboard for long periods of time. You may experience considerable frustration if you do not recover in the expected amount of time and can no longer perform your job. If you feel guilty or blamed for not returning to work, you may become angry at your employers for not setting up the computer correctly in the first place.

These feelings are often made worse by the lack of caring shown for a worker's physical and emotional needs. Although worker's compensation was originally designed as a sort of no-fault insurance for employers and their employees, this is rarely the case when chronic pain conditions occur. Once again, legal involvement may serve to delay resolution or to assign blame when actually none exists. Assigning blame may be appropriate in cases of harm resulting from negligence, accidents, or assault; it may not always be possible in cases of chronic pain. If you are a pain patient in such circumstances, it is important to avoid assigning blame inappropriately (to either yourself or others) and to realize that you can move on to the next phase.

Phase 4: Balancing the Scales. When the need to take responsibility for coping with the injury has been admitted (Phase 2), and the question of whom, if anyone, needs to be held responsible for causing the injury has been resolved (Phase 3), then forgiving can proceed. Forgiving begins from a position of strength. If you continue to feel powerless to cope with your pain, then anger may keep you a victim. Accepting the responsibility to *live with* the pain, as opposed to responsibility for *causing* the pain, can empower you. Coping is best done from a position of self-awareness. If you are aware of your feelings and motivations, you can identify where your responsibilities end and those of others begin, thus balancing the scale.

When an injurer is found to be responsible, then punishment through the courts and restitution, not revenge or recrimination, is in order. This was probably the original role of the legal system in such circumstances.

Phase 5: Choosing to Forgive. The art of forgiving implies that you are ready to let go of the negative feelings that until now have imprisoned your mind, spirit, and heart. In so doing, you move toward repairing the injury by moving on with the life you have now. Forgiveness is coming to accept your new life, even if it is one of pain. Through this process, forgivers find and create new answers that, in a way, make them new people. "If nothing can ever be the same, this time around, perhaps it can be better" (Flanigan, 1992, p. 162).

Writing the Wrongs

The writing exercise mentioned in the "Exploration Tasks" of Chapter 5 has been helpful to people who have trouble identifying the thoughts and reasons behind their anger. Begin by asking yourself, "Who has hurt me and what have they done?" Then list what you gain by staying angry and what you gain by giving up your anger. Compare the two sides of your list. What are your conclusions?

Healthy Attitudes

Much research focuses on negative attitudes and their relationship to ill health. However, some researchers have identified attitudes that go with positive health.

Stress Hardiness

Suzanne Kobasa of the University of Chicago studied "stress-hardy" executives. These were people who viewed life changes as challenges rather than as threats; they felt committed to their work, as well as to their families and social institutions. They also believed that their response to whatever happened was within their control. The research found that they experienced fewer physical and emotional symptoms during a particularly stressful business period than those without these qualities.

Another researcher who has examined positive health attitudes is Aaron Antonovsky of the Ben-Gurion University of the Negev in Israel. Antonovsky talked with a group of Holocaust survivors in Israel who appeared to have remained in good emotional health in spite of their having experienced terrible trauma. From his discussions with these exceptional survivors and others, Antonovsky has gone on to develop his theory of the "sense of coherence." He has proposed that people with a high sense of coherence have a pervasive, enduring, yet dynamic feeling of confidence that (1) stressors coming from the internal and external environments are structured, predictable, and explicable; (2) they themselves have resources available to meet the demands resulting from these stressors; and (3) these demands are challenges worthy of investment and engagement.

Optimism

Optimism, too, has been declared a healthy attitude. Optimists are people who expect things to turn out well; they expect to enjoy life. Optimism has been associated with an enhanced immune system. Sandra Levy, a psychoneuroimmunologist, has shown that an optimistic explanatory style strongly predicts the length of cancer remission (see Karren et al. in "Supplementary Reading"). Martin Seligman has demonstrated that a pessimistic style is associated with depression and general poor health. Pessimists see events that happen to them as stable ("This *always* happens to me"), global ("I *never* do anything right"), and internal ("It's all *my* fault"). In contrast, optimists see events as unstable ("Just because it happened once doesn't mean it will again"), specific ("I have trouble with pacing my work activities"), and external ("Other people are responsible for their behaviors, I'm responsible for mine").

Empathy

There are several definitions of the word "empathy." Here, I mean a *nonjudgmental* awareness of others' experience. Remember the excerpt from Joan's writing exercise at the beginning of Chapter 5? If you were able to come to some understanding of what Joan was experiencing, you were feeling empathy. On the other hand, if you found yourself making critical or unflattering comments, then you were judging.

Judgment is in order when we assess the content of our own thoughts. But many times we are too quick to judge others. We can be wrong, for example, in deciding that a person has no redeeming qualities. We may cut off our chance to explore further explanations or possibilities. We can have a strong tendency to make quick judgments when we are feeling out of control.

Suspending judgment may at first seem too open-ended. You may fear it requires you to remain in an eternal state of ambiguity. Actually, it gives you the time necessary to gather information, to walk in the other person's shoes, and to experience various viewpoints. It asks you to be patient for others and ultimately for yourself. We base many of our judgments on illusions and misinformation; we only *think* we know what's going on much of the time. It's okay to relax about the long process necessary for change. Suspend the tendency to evaluate your efforts as good or bad, right or wrong. Explore the wide range of possibilities and choices that lie before you. Such flexibility is a key to the positive attitudes that can enhance your health and life.

Altruism

> A rabbi had a conversation with the Lord about Heaven and Hell. "I will show you Hell," said the Lord, and led the rabbi into a room in the middle of which was a very big round table. The people sitting at it were starving and desperate.
>
> In the middle of the room was an enormous pot of stew, more than enough for everyone. The smell of the stew was delicious and made the rabbi's mouth water. The people around the table were holding spoons with very long handles. Each person found that it was just possible to reach the pot to take a spoonful of the stew, but because the handle of the spoon was longer than anyone's arm, no one could get the food into his mouth.
>
> The rabbi saw that their suffering was indeed terrible. "Now I will show you Heaven," said the Lord, and they went into another room which was exactly the same as the first room. There was the same big round table and the same enormous pot of stew. The people, as before, were equipped with the same long-handled spoons. But here they were well nourished and plump, laughing, and talking.
>
> At first the rabbi could not understand. "It is simple, but requires a certain skill," said the Lord. "You see, they have learned to feed each other." (Jewish folk tale)*

We need each other. Nurturing this connectedness can be very difficult when you are in pain, because pain can preoccupy you to such an extent that it shuts your eyes to the needs of others. Once you have established what kind of pacing of activities you require, think seriously about joining a support group, volunteering, or get-

---

*Retold by Irvin D. Yalom in *The Theory and Practice of Group Psychotherapy, Third Edition* (New York: Basic Books, 1975, pp. 12–13).

ting involved with a political passion you may have, so as to help fulfill someone else's needs.

Building a Foundation for Attitude Change

> Assume a virtue, though you have it not. . . . Refrain tonight;
> And that shall lend a kind of easiness to the next abstinence:
>   the next more easy;
> For practice can almost change the stamp of nature.
> —*William Shakespeare*, Hamlet

If you don't already have them, you can develop healthier attitudes such as stress hardiness, optimism, empathy, and altruism. Attitudes are not fixed or unchangeable. It is possible to change the filters through which you see your world.

The following techniques will help you develop healthier attitudes. Affirmations can encourage your positive self-talk and nurture your self-esteem, examining the sources of your self-esteem can help strengthen your courage and fortitude, and humor can ease the hard work of change.

Affirmations

You can use affirmations to change your attitudes in a positive way. Affirmations are short positive statements, quotes, or reflections that you can repeat to yourself. They make you feel inspired, comforted, or supported.

There are many ways of developing and using affirmations. You may find inspiration in a book that provides daily reflections (for example, see Schaef in "Supplementary Reading") or in spiritual books. Or you may select a quote, phrase, or passage that simply comes to mind during the day's activities. You may find that an affirmation comes to you at the end of an RR technique (see Chapter 3). You may not always agree at first with this spontaneous affirmation, but if you repeat it throughout the day, you may find that it inspires you to consider a feeling or attitude you wish to develop.

For example, you may end your RR technique with the statement "I am strong." It arises from your unconscious, but your more conscious self says, "Who are you kidding? I don't feel strong at all! I'm the original 120-pound weakling!" As you repeat the affirmation "I am strong" periodically for a week, however, you may begin to appreciate that you are getting in touch with qualities of strength that are not physical in nature. That is, you are developing strength through courage, fortitude, and will. You feel inspired to do more with your life as a result. Often, the most useful and relevant affirmations are those you generate yourself.

Write out a few affirmations that come to you during the next week while you are practicing an RR technique. Post them on the refrigerator or on the dashboard of your car so that you can be reminded of them. See what happens.

Examining the Sources of Self-Esteem

Self-esteem, or the way you feel about yourself, is the end result of many factors. The DAS (see Chapter 5) can help you to identify the unchallenged assumptions that make adapting to life more difficult. The following exercise can also help you strengthen your vulnerable areas.

Write 10 things that you like about yourself:

1. _____
2. _____
3. _____
4. _____
5. _____
6. _____
7. _____
8. _____
9. _____
10. _____

Now, write 10 things that you don't like about yourself or would like to change:

1. _____
2. _____
3. _____
4. _____
5. _____
6. _____
7. _____
8. _____
9. _____
10. _____

Which list was easier to complete? _____ Why? _____

_____

_____

If you're like most people, the negative things come more easily to mind. Saying what you like about yourself is often labeled as conceited or self-centered, so you may feel compelled to qualify positive statements with "but" or "not always." Remember: It's okay to feel satisfied with something you do, feel, or like about yourself.

Look at the list that contains things you like about yourself. Put a check mark (✓) next to those things that are internal characteristics ("patience," "compassionate," "good listener"). Put an (x) next to those characteristics that are external ("good worker," "good friend," "pretty face"). Is there a balance of (✓) and (x), or are you heavy on the (x) side?

Traits that are external are more vulnerable to the judgments of others and to losses (such as loss of job, good health, or personal relations). Many people in pain suffer even more when their major source of self-esteem resides in what they do (or did) for a career. It's important for people to have both internal and external qualities on which to build their self-esteem. It creates a firm foundation for engaging with the world.

See whether you can balance your list of positive traits with both external and internal attributes. Are there any traits on your negative list that you might turn into positive traits through goal setting?

Humor

Just as people with pain tend to lose self-esteem, they can also lose the ability to see the humor or joy in themselves and in the world around them. The preoccupation with self and the sadness of losing "normal" abilities can make humor or joy difficult to find. The ability to use humor or find joy in life promotes a healthier interaction of mind and body that does not require you to be pain free.

In Chapter 5, you may have found yourself chuckling while identifying your automatic thoughts. You may have wondered, "Now where in the world did I get *that* idea?!" Laughing at your own follies and foibles is healthy. It can generate positive attitudes that last long after the laugh. It insures flexibility and reminds you not to take everything so seriously. In fact, laughter is thought to enhance the production of endorphins (the body's natural opiates), which can diminish pain awareness.

However, some humor, especially wisecracking, can be used to hide underlying negative attitudes that need to be explored. Good-natured deliberate giggling, on the other hand, is not only desirable, it is necessary. It's also important to be able to laugh spontaneously. Indeed, the way real life challenges our assumptions and expectations is often the source of our biggest laughs.

If you are finding it hard to find something to laugh about, watch a funny movie; read a favorite book of cartoons; read the writings of Loretta Laroche or other astute life observers; buy a joke book; or, if you really get stuck, watch small children at play. Somehow, adulthood becomes "a-dolt-hood" for too many of us. Commit yourself now to consciously seeking out a giggle, if not an outright guffaw, on at least a weekly basis.

Summary

- Changing negative lifestyles, behaviors, and attitudes provides specific health benefits and can greatly improve your ability to cope with chronic pain.

- An attitude is a psychological characteristic that results from many influences. It is generally adopted without thinking.

- Holding on to certain negative attitudes can impair health and prevent flexibility in new circumstances. Such attitudes need to be examined consciously.

- Learned helplessness can paralyze you to such an extent that you cannot work on healing. Remember that you do have choices and you do have control.

- Anger has a place, but holding on to it is destructive. Forgiveness is one way of coping effectively with anger; there are five phases for forgiveness.

- Stress-hardy and optimistic people are healthier and cope better with stress.

- Empathy is a nonjudgmental understanding of what someone is feeling; it can help you avoid rash decisions and can increase your options.

- Altruism is an important way of staying connected with others.

- Affirmations are short, positive statements, quotes, or reflections that you can repeat to yourself for inspiration, comfort, or support.

- Self-esteem is how you feel about yourself. Most people find it easier to get in touch with their negative qualities than with their positive ones; however, remembering your positive traits will enhance your self-esteem.

- Conscious humor is healthy. It is associated with the production of endorphins and generates positive attitudes that last long after the laugh.

Exploration Tasks

1. Continue recording your automatic thoughts associated with negative emotional states (see Chapter 5). Identify the distortions and their possible sources through your own explorations. Change the automatic thoughts to reflect the reality of the situation, using any of the three reframing techniques discussed in Chapter 5. Copy and use the worksheet at the back of the book to record your explorations in negative self-talk. As you employ the techniques suggested in the present chapter, do you find your self-talk becoming more positive?

2. Continue with your practice of the basic RR techniques (1–5) on a daily basis. As suggested in the text, use phrases and statements that come to you during your RR practice as personal affirmations.

3. Write out a goal that you want to accomplish related to the material in this chapter. As

always, make sure your goal is a behavioral task that you can measure in terms of the steps *you* will take to accomplish it. Here is an example:

Goal: *To do something that makes me laugh at least once a week.*

Steps to take to reach that goal:

A. *Read The New Yorker.*

B. *Rent a humorous video.*

C. *Read the newspaper cartoons.*

Now it's your turn.

Goal: _____

Steps to take to reach that goal:

A. _____

B. _____

C. _____

D. _____

In addition, list contingency plans. That is, identify what obstacles might get in the way of your accomplishing this goal. What solutions can you devise to work toward insuring the success of this goal?

	Obstacles	**Solutions**
A.	_____	_____
B.	_____	_____
C.	_____	_____
D.	_____	_____

Supplementary Reading

The following books provide additional information on attitudes and how to change them:

Fawzy I. Fawzy, Nancy Fawzy, Christine Hyun, Robert Elashoff, Donald Guthrie, John Fahey, et al., "Malignant Melanoma: Effects of an Early Structured Psychiatric Intervention, Coping, and Affective State on Recurrence and Survival 6 Years Later," *Archives of General Psychiatry*, 50: 681–688, 1993.

Beverly Flanigan, *Forgiving the Unforgivable: Overcoming the Bitter Legacy of Intimate Wounds* (New York: Wiley, 1992).

Keith K. Karren, Brent Q. Hafen, Kathryn J. Frandsen, and Lee Smith, *Mind/Body Health:*

Effects of Attitudes, Emotions and Relationships, Third Edition. (Boston: Benjamin Cummings, 2006).

Jeff Keller, *Attitude Is Everything* (Tampa, FL: International Network Training Institute, 2007).

Allen Klein, *The Healing Power of Humor* (Los Angeles: Tarcher, 1989).

Suzanne Kobasa, "Stressful Life Events, Personality and Health: An Inquiry into Hardiness," *Journal of Personality and Social Psychology, 37:* 1–11, 1979.

Loretta Laroche, *Life Is Not a Stress Rehearsal: Bringing Yesterday's Sane Wisdom into Today's Insane World* (New York: Broadway Books, 2001).

Miriam Nelson, Wendy Wray, and Sarah Wernick, *Strong Women Stay Young* (New York: Bantam, 2005).

Robert Ornstein and David Sobel, *Healthy Pleasures* (New York: Da Capo Press, 1990).

Anne Wilson Schaef, *Meditations for Women Who Do Too Much, Revised Edition* (San Francisco: HarperOne, 2004).

Niall Scott and Jonathan Seglow, *Altruism* (New York: Open University Press, 2007).

Martin Seligman, *Learned Optimism: How to Change Your Mind and Your Life* (New York: Vintage, 2006).

Idries Shah, *The Pleasantries of the Incredible Mulla Nasrudin* (London: Octagon Press, 1983).

Idries Shah, *Reflections* (London: Octagon Press, 1983).

Idries Shah, *The Subtleties of the Inimitable Mulla Nasrudin* and *The Exploits of the Incomparable Mulla Nasrudin* (London: Octagon Press, 1989).

Redford B. Williams and Virginia Williams, *Anger Kills: Seventeen Strategies for Controlling the Hostility That Can Harm Your Health* (New York: Harper Paperbacks, 1998).

Denise Winn, *The Manipulated Mind: Brainwashing, Conditioning and Manipulation* (Los Altos, CA: Malor Books, 2000).

7

Nutrition and Pain

Why Discuss Nutrition?

Why include a chapter on nutrition in a pain management book? Well, there are three reasons. First, good eating habits are essential for good health; the program described in this book treats the whole person, as well as the pain. Second, some specific foods and eating behaviors can affect pain levels (these are discussed in more detail later). Third, there is a great deal of misinformation at present about nutritional therapies for pain. This last point deserves additional comment.

The United States as a culture is obsessed with diets, body weight, and food; few Americans consider eating simply as basic sustenance. Food is everywhere and food remedies, diets, and supplements are eagerly adopted by the public. There has also been a growing dissatisfaction with organized medicine, particularly in treating chronic disease. Patients are increasingly willing to embrace such "natural," "holistic" therapies as megadose vitamin therapy, fasting, and internal cleansing. The language used to justify the claims for some of these nutritional treatments sounds scientific, but there is rarely evidence other than personal testimonials to support their claims.

Here are just some of the difficulties encountered in studies of nutritional therapies, which are the reasons that such studies must be designed and evaluated carefully. An examination of research papers on the process of digestion and absorption of food components makes it apparent that the whole process of nutrition is not a simple one. For example, some food components are only absorbed when needed by the body, and others are absorbed only if there are other essential components available in the same meal. Add to that the complexity of asking every single participant in a nutritional study to eat the same thing while meeting individual metabolic needs for a long enough time to see changes in symptoms, and you can see that the task is formidable.

Rheumatoid arthritis is the most common pain syndrome studied for dietary influences. The research has involved three lines of investigation: fish and plant oils, vegetarian/fasting diets, and hypersensitivity/food allergies. The strongest evidence supports the intake of fish oils that contain omega-3 polyunsaturated fatty acids, but even these studies are not definitive. Fish oil has not been shown to benefit osteoarthritis. Plant oils thought to promote anti-inflammatory effects are flaxseed oil (1 to 3 tablespoons per day), a source of eicosapentaenoic acid (EPA), and evening primrose and borage oils, sources of gamma-linoleic acid (GLA), at up to 2,800 mgs per day. WARNING: The amounts of these specific fatty acids needed for them to be effective can also interfere with blood clotting. Check with your doctor if you are planning to take these supplements and are on anti-inflammatory drugs or blood-thinning drugs (for example, Coumadin®), or using ginger or turmeric.

The other investigations have produced mixed results regarding dietary effects on symptoms of rheumatoid arthritis. The most that can and should be said at this time about special diets is that some people with rheumatoid arthritis appear to benefit from eliminating dairy products; reducing saturated fats, which are higher in nonvegetarian diets; and eliminating certain foods, like wheat, corn, peanuts, or eggs, and some food additives or seasonings, such as MSG (monosodium glutamate). Elimination diets to test food sensitivities are complicated to institute and should be undertaken with the supervision of a dietitian and/or doctor who is experienced in such diets. See "Supplementary Reading" for more detailed references on these topics.

In the other chronic pain syndromes, there is no firm evidence that food allergies play a role or that improvements can be obtained with extreme dietary supplementation (for example, megadoses of vitamins or minerals or extracts of animal hormones and herbs) or elimination (for example, yeast-free diets). In other words, there is simply not enough proof that such treatments work to recommend them. Indeed, there is often potential harm with such treatments. The harm can include dietary deficiencies, imbalances, and toxicities, as well as enormous financial costs to patients. I do endorse the careful study of nutritional therapies. I also recommend keeping an open mind to the possibility that in the future some patients will be able to control their pain symptoms with dietary manipulation.

In the interim, while we're all awaiting further clarification, you can begin following some basic nutritional recommendations now to improve your general health and help you in your pain management. These are explored in the following pages.

Two Important Principles

I summarize my basic approach to nutrition in the following two slogans: "Fresh is best" and "Moderation." It may be more difficult than you think to follow these two simple recommendations. Prepared, processed, and fast foods are widely available, the frantic pace of life leaves little time for meal preparation, and many people in pain get a soothing feeling from eating.

"Fresh is best" because foods prepared by others are more likely to have added salt, sugar, saturated fats, preservatives, and artificial coloring. Much of this manipulation of food is the result of processing foods to give them a longer shelf life. These foods also tend to appeal to the average American consumer, who has been eating a diet high in fat and sodium and low in fiber for quite a while. However, increased processing may decrease fiber and nutritional content. There is also increasing evidence that low-fiber, high-fat, and high-sodium diets may put individuals at risk for developing heart disease, some cancers (colon cancer), high blood pressure, and obesity. America is facing an obesity epidemic that is increasing at an alarming rate. Obesity can increase the risk of diabetes and degenerative joint disease (osteoarthritis), particularly in the lower extremities; this is of particular concern to people already experiencing chronic pain, as it can complicate the pain management problem further.

By "moderation" I mean eating that results in a stable weight, appropriate for your height and body type. Eat at regular times, from a variety of foods in the four basic food groups (discussed below). Eat in quantities that meet the caloric requirements of your activities and metabolism. This will help you maintain a stable weight. Skipping meals, eating your largest meal in the evening, and snacking on high-fat foods (chips, ice cream, cakes, or candy) contribute to weight problems. If not overwhelmed by excess, the body appears to have a natural wisdom that enables it to pick and choose what it needs, when it needs it.

Basic Nutritional Guidelines

The typical American diet contributes to increases in obesity, diabetes, heart disease, and stroke. Over the past decade, the U.S. Department of Agriculture (USDA), the U.S. Department of Health and Human Services, and the American Heart Association have made recommendations for changing what we eat. The USDA food pyramid released in 2005 recommends not only what to eat but also in what amounts. If you go to the website (*www.mypyramid.gov*), you can get a personalized diet recommendation based on your age, height, weight, and exercise level. An alternative approach is offered by Harvard's School of Public Health. Its Healthy Eating Pyramid, which can be found at *www.hsph.harvard.edu/nutritionsource*, offers nutritional information based on the best evidence available. It can also tell you about food pyramid history and politics. The Oldways Preservation and Exchange Trust offers good, evidence-based guides for healthy eating from other cultures and vegetarianism. You can find its website at *www.oldwayspt.org*.

The most recent recommendations encourage a diet that reduces portion amounts, saturated fats, and cholesterol, and so reduces weight. Let's take a look.

1. *Portion amounts.* Picture a dinner plate that is divided in half. One half of the plate represents the amount of fruits and vegetables you should eat. One quarter of the plate area is the recommended portion of meat or meat substitute (the size of a deck of cards), and the other quarter is the whole grains/starch portion. Research shows that portion size at restau-

rants increased between 1977 and 1996, with the largest increases at fast-food places. The increased portions meant increased calories from foods lower in nutritional value. The website *hp2010.nhlbihin.net/portion/servingcard7.pdf* has a serving portion reference card. Print it and laminate it to help you with portion control.

2. *Healthy eating.* Include a variety of fruits, vegetables, whole grains, legumes (beans), fish, lean meat, and poultry in your diet. Each day eat a variety of vegetables, fruits, and grain products (make whole grains at least half of the grains you consume). Eat lean meats, fish (one to two 6-ounce servings/week), nuts, and beans as a source of protein. Use fat-free and low-fat dairy products.

3. *Weight loss (and maintaining a normal weight).* Weight loss helps protect the weight-bearing joints from deterioration, but it is also important for a healthy lifestyle. To lose weight you must eat *fewer* calories than you burn. So, you can increase activities to burn more calories—aerobic exercise and strengthening (resistance training) exercises—or decrease your calorie intake.

Other ways to eat healthy and lose weight include reducing or eliminating sweet soft drinks and commercially prepared baked goods, and increasing exercise to 30 minutes a day of brisk walking or comparable activity or at least 180 minutes per week of combined activity/exercise. Resistance training is a good way to increase metabolism. Use 3- to 5-pound weights every other day to do up to three sets of 12 repetitions each with five to six muscle groups. You may need professional guidance if you have been inactive for a while. And if so, start with 1-pound weights and fewer repetitions. If you have any questions talk with your physician or physical therapist or a personal trainer who is familiar with chronic pain.

Plan on a gradual weight loss of 1 to 2 pounds per week. Although this may seem slow, it will help keep the weight off in the end. Remember: it's easier to prevent obesity than to lose weight. Follow the recommendations for healthy diet, activity, and portion size before you develop a weight problem.

Basic Food Group Nutrients

The six basic food groups are:

- Grains (whole and refined)
- Vegetables
- Fruits
- Milk, yogurt, and cheese
- Meat, poultry, fish, dry beans, eggs, and nuts
- Oils

They provide us with the following nutrients:

- Carbohydrates
- Proteins
- Fats
- Vitamins and minerals

Carbohydrates

Carbohydrates are either simple or complex. Simple carbohydrates are sugars, such as table sugar, honey, and syrups. Use simple sugars in small amounts. Sugar has a bad reputation in U.S. culture, but the main problem for adults is the company it keeps, such as the fat in pastries and ice cream. Eating fresh fruit can satisfy a sweet tooth and is a healthier choice.

Complex carbohydrates are made up of repeating chains of sugar molecules. Starch is an example of a complex carbohydrate. Vegetables and grains are excellent sources of complex carbohydrates, as well as of fiber, vitamins, and iron. The way the digestive system absorbs carbohydrates can be difficult to predict. To help, a new guideline, *the glycemic index,* was developed. This index classifies carbohydrates by how quickly they are absorbed and how much they increase blood sugar compared to pure glucose. Foods with a high glycemic index, like sugar-sweetened beverages, cause rapid spikes in blood sugar. Foods with soluble fiber (such as whole grains: cracked wheat, oatmeal, brown rice) generally have a low glycemic index. For example, whole oats are digested slowly, causing a lower and more gradual change in blood sugar. Foods with a score of 70 or higher are defined as having a high glycemic index; those with a score of 55 or below have a low glycemic index. You can search for the glycemic index rating of more than 1,000 carbohydrates by going to *www.glycemicindex.com,* sponsored by the University of Sydney (Australia).

Proteins

Proteins are made up of amino acid units, which are used by the body after being broken down in digestion; they are either metabolized for energy or reassembled into new proteins. Proteins are the building blocks of enzymes, hormones, and muscle tissue. Meat, poultry, fish, dry beans, eggs, and nuts are good sources of protein. Meat as a food source is inherently good, but it has fallen into disrepute because it can contain a lot of hormones and antibiotics (given to animals while alive), it is a source of saturated fat and cholesterol, and in the past it was associated with diets of little nutritional variety ("meat and potatoes"). In addition, for a variety of reasons (including religious convictions, the rising financial and ecological costs of meat, and growing sensitivity to animal rights), increasing numbers of people are choosing to reduce their meat intake.

Fats

Fats are made up of substances called "fatty acids" and "glycerol. " Fatty acids can be saturated, polyunsaturated, or monounsaturated; the less saturated they are, the healthier they are. Glycerol is the "carrier" that binds fatty acids together. Fats are used for energy and are easily stored in the body, and we all know their favorite storage places—the thighs, abdomen, and buttocks.

As mentioned earlier, some fatty acids turn into inflammatory products. Known as omega-6 linoleic fatty acids, they are commonly found in corn and safflower oil, and converted to arachidonic acids that then form "bad" leukotrienes and prostaglandins, which cause inflammation. The omega-3 linoleic fatty acids found in fish oils, flaxseed, and soybeans contain EPA and DHA, which help form the "good" prostaglandins and leukotrienes that reduce inflammation. If your chronic pain has an inflammation component, consider changing your balance of omega-3 fatty acids and omega-6 fatty acids. It may be helpful. Even if your pain is not due to inflammation, there is evidence that changes in the types of fatty acids you eat can help your heart and may help prevent some cancers. For example, avoid trans fats (hydrogenated fats like shortening or stick margarine).

The best source of fish oils is cold-water fish (sardines, trout, salmon). Capsules of fish oil, borage, and evening primrose oil (that contain gamma-linoleic acid) are available to supplement the diet. But you have to take large numbers of capsules a day to change your fatty acid balance; the expense may be prohibitive. Remember to check with your physician if you are on blood thinners and choose to supplement with the omega-3 oils. As with many dietary recommendations, it may be better to alter what you eat to include the foods recommended for healthy eating than to depend on supplements in an unhealthy diet.

Cholesterol is not a fat; it is a substance present in some foods, such as eggs, dairy products, and animal fats (always animal products). The intake of fat and cholesterol in the diet contributes to the body's production of cholesterol. This is the reason you hear the terms "cholesterol" and "fats" together so often. There are several types of cholesterol, and too much cholesterol of one type (low-density lipoprotein, or LDL) can contribute to diseases such as atherosclerosis (hardening of the arteries) and gallstones.

Vitamins and Minerals

Vitamins and minerals are food elements necessary in very small amounts for the body's normal functioning. They are essential in our diet because the body can't make them or makes them in insufficient amounts. Vegetables and grains are good sources of vitamins. There is considerable controversy regarding the benefit of vitamin and mineral supplements in health and disease. For a normal healthy adult, eating a variety of foods should provide the essential nutrients; the body can choose what it needs, when needed. No research has disputed this to date. What are the needs of a stressed or ill body? I consider this question next.

Managing Pain through Nutrition

> What is food to one, is to others bitter poison.
> —*Lucretius (circa 94–55 B.C.)*

The information presented above should guide your basic nutrition, but there is room for a great deal of individual variation. Everyone has different digestive and metabolic rates, genetic compositions, and activity levels. All of this affects food requirements. Be cautious about the many conflicting and sometimes dangerous diet fads. The two pain syndromes that have received the most attention in terms of food-related symptom worsening are rheumatoid arthritis, discussed earlier, and migraine headaches.

Again, there does appear to be an internal body wisdom. You can learn from your body if you do not ignore its signals, such as increasing pain, fatigue, or indigestion after eating certain foods or drinking certain beverages. Just as you should learn to listen to your pain and distress, listen to your body's response to eating. This will help you to understand how you eat, when you eat, what you eat, and why you eat.

Certain foods and beverages are associated with increased pain in some people. Keep a food diary similar to your pain diary (one is provided at the back of the book). Use it to identify patterns. For example, do you avoid certain drinks or foods because of your pain? If so, what do you avoid? Do you eat more of a certain food group? If so, what foods are these?

How to Eat: Behavioral "Appetizers" and "Desserts"

We live in a fast-paced, high-stress society. For those who have the added challenge of pain, it is particularly important to take the proper time to prepare to eat.

Before you begin your meal, take a few moments to smell the aromas and look at the colors of the food before you. Saying grace or giving thanks may be a way to allow you to pause in this manner before taking your nourishment.

Try, when possible, to eat without distractions. Avoid eating with a newspaper, a magazine, or the television in front of you. Notice what it feels like just to eat. Are you bored or anxious? Does eating feel pleasurable?

After eating, take a few moments to read, enjoy a pleasurable activity, or daydream as your body digests its food. If you feel uncomfortable or bloated, or have indigestion, it may reflect what you've eaten or how you've eaten. These are important cues to document in your diary.

When to Eat

Many of us eat on an uneven or arbitrary schedule. Some people eat between meals because those are the times they find themselves hungry or bored. Others skip meals and consume most of their calories in the evening.

We have known for a long time that eating a good breakfast (literally, "breakfast") is a healthy thing to do; it supplies your body with the energy to start your daily activities. Skipping breakfast leads to bad nutritional habits, such as grabbing doughnuts, candy, or soft drinks later in the morning. If people who are prone to hypoglycemia (low blood sugar) do this, they will experience mood swings, irritability, and increased pain. The discomfort can be relieved by sweets—only to recur with even greater intensity several hours later.

People with a family history of diabetes may have hypoglycemia but this is not always the case. Many physicians deny that the condition exists or has any discernable symptoms, though glucose tolerance tests can document its presence. It is worsened by prolonged fasting periods. Susceptible people find that when they eat sweets in isolation as described above, they experience symptoms an hour or two later that are thought to be due to low blood sugar. In addition to the mood symptoms noted above, shakiness, sweating, headaches, muscle aches, and fatigue may result. Snack on fruit or yogurt instead of candy bars, and eat small, frequent meals, thus avoiding prolonged periods of fasting. A number of patients with headaches and fibromyalgia have found that their symptoms improved after they followed these recommendations.

Eating the largest meal of the day in the evening is not conducive to using the nutrients for energy. It may contribute to weight gain, poor sleep, and reflux (the movement of acid from the stomach back into the esophagus) if sleep follows too closely after the evening meal.

What to Eat and Why

Once again, eating a variety of fresh foods in moderation is the key to healthy eating. If you need to lose weight, watch the fat content of your foods, exercise, and consume moderate portions.

Identifying what you eat and noting any corresponding increase or decrease in your pain can also help you determine which foods, ingredients, or additives to avoid and which foods to keep in your diet. (Some specific suggestions are provided below.)

Identifying why you eat is also critical, because many people who have pain report that eating makes them feel good, at least temporarily. Eating is thought to release endorphins (the body's own painkillers), which may explain this good feeling. So considering how eating makes you feel may give you important clues to getting the most out of your diet. You may find, for instance, that you overeat for comfort. Nurturing yourself in other ways—through practicing RR techniques, becoming aware of other pleasurable activities, and seeking social support—may help reduce your need for "comfort eating."

Food Ingredients/Additives Linked to Increased Pain

Let's take a look at the following culprits that have been associated with increases in pain:

- Caffeine

- Alcohol

- Monosodium glutamate (MSG)

- Aspartame

Caffeine. Caffeine is an addictive stimulant, so it is advisable to consider decreasing your caffeine intake when you are under a lot of stress or in pain. But be careful: You can experience headaches and fatigue if you suddenly stop drinking caffeinated beverages altogether. Instead of stopping abruptly, you should gradually decrease your intake to avoid withdrawal symptoms. For example, instead of having five cups of coffee each morning, try two cups of decaffeinated coffee and three cups of regular coffee for a week. Next, continue to decrease the number of cups of regular coffee until you are drinking only decaffeinated coffee. Then decrease the number of cups of decaf as well, if you wish.

Caffeine is naturally present in coffee, tea, chocolate, and cocoa. It is also found in some soft drinks (such as colas and energy drinks) and in many prescription and nonprescription drugs (particularly cold, pain, stimulant, and weight-control preparations). The following table shows how caffeine levels can vary, depending on the type of beverage and how it is prepared.

Caffeine Content of Common Beverages

Beverage	Measure	Caffeine (mg)
Coffee		
Brewed, ground	8 ounces	80–200*
Instant	1 teaspoon	50–66
Decaffeinated	1 teaspoon	2–5
Tea (regular bag)		20–100*
Brewed 3 minutes		36
Brewed 5 minutes		46
Soft drinks		
Colas	12 ounces	43–65
Hot cocoa	8 ounces	5–10

*The longer the coffee and tea are brewed, the greater the caffeine content.

Alcohol. Alcohol is a blood vessel dilator and therefore may trigger migraines or worsen existing headaches. An earlier theory that migraines were caused by blood vessel dilatation following intense constriction is now known to be inaccurate or at best inadequate. However, some migraine sufferers find that alcohol is best left alone, whatever the underlying mechanism may be. Other substances that may dilate blood vessels are tyramine and histamine. Tyramine can be found in red wine and some cheeses; histamine can be found in some wines and champagnes. (See the article by Radnitz in "Supplementary Reading.")

Many other people with pain also find a link between pain and alcohol use. If you do *not* find that your pain improves when alcohol is eliminated from your diet, then drinking in moderation is best. If you *do* find that your pain improves when alcohol is eliminated, you would do well to avoid alcohol completely.

Remember that alcoholic beverages also contain a lot of calories. One and a half ounces of gin, rum, vodka, or whiskey contain about 116 calories. A 12-ounce can of beer has about 145 calories.

Using alcohol to numb pain can be a problem. Although it is an age-old remedy for acute pain, its use in chronic pain can create more physical and social problems in the long run. If you drink alcohol within 2 hours of bedtime, it can disrupt your sleep. It reduces the deep sleep and dreaming stages. Excessive drinking can also result in liver, pancreas, muscle, and brain dysfunction in susceptible individuals. If you have ever felt that you should cut down on your drinking, ever been annoyed by people criticizing your drinking, ever felt bad or guilty about your drinking, or ever had a drink first thing in the morning to steady your nerves or get rid of a hangover, then it would be wise to take heed and seek medical help.

MSG. MSG is a flavor enhancer found in many prepared foods but commonly associated with Chinese food. Individuals sensitive to MSG may experience headaches, a burning sensation in the face, sweating, and chest tightness. Studies show that people who experience migraines may or may not be more prone to headaches caused by MSG. Avoidance is the best treatment if you are sensitive. But beware: MSG can be hidden in broth or bouillon cubes and other food products, so read labels to determine whether it is present.

Aspartame. Aspartame (brand name: NutraSweet®) has been associated with headache symptoms in sensitive individuals. Aspartame can be found in a wide assortment of diet products; again, check the labels. If you are drinking a lot of diet drinks or eating a lot of diet products that contain aspartame, you may want to stop consuming them to see whether there is any effect on your pain, especially if you are experiencing headaches.

The Role of Vitamins and Minerals in Reducing Pain

The use of magnesium, zinc, B vitamins, and vitamins E and C has been promoted in chronic pain conditions that have an inflammatory component. The lack of consistent scientific findings may reflect human variability and the subjective nature of pain rather than the failure of these supplements to help. On the other hand, this may mean these supplements have no value. At this time, there is no consistent evidence that taking most mineral or vitamin supplements (in addition to your normal diet) is helpful in relieving pain.

A calcium-rich diet or calcium supplementation is important, however, because of the high incidence of osteoporosis (brittle bones) in postmenopausal women and in men as well, although they develop the condition 5 to 10 years later. Vitamin D is also important because of its role in bone formation. Adequate amounts of this vitamin may be obtained through supplemented milk or exposure to sunlight below the 40th latitude. Above the 40th latitude, that is, above San Francisco, Denver, or Philadelphia, the winter sun exposure is not adequate. Osteoporosis is the number one cause of disability in women over 65 years of age in the United States and is associated with fractures of the spine and hip. Men and women both start losing calcium from their bone stores in their 30s; after menopause, however, the rate of loss for susceptible women is accelerated. Risk factors include the following:

- Having a family history of osteoporosis
- Being white and of northern European background
- Smoking
- Being thin
- Being inactive

There has been a lot of controversy regarding how much calcium women should take and in what form. For prevention, current recommendations encourage women to get an adequate amount of calcium in their diet before menopause. The dosage recommended is 1,000 milligrams per day of calcium for nonpregnant, nonlactating women over 25 years of age. This dosage is equal to four 8-ounce glasses of milk or five Tums® tablets a day. For postmenopausal women who are at risk for osteoporosis, the recommended dosage is 1,200 milligrams of calcium per day. The association of increased coronary artery disease with calcium supplementation in older women has recently been reported. This will need further observation and future study. Other sources of calcium are yogurt and other dairy products, and green leafy vegetables. Regular exercise also helps with prevention. There are also medications available to treat osteoporosis, for example, Fosamax®, Miacalcin®, and Evista®. Caution is needed if bisphosphonates (such as Fosamax®) are prescribed because of recent reports of severe musculoskeletal pain and rare jawbone pain.

Summary

Why Discuss Nutrition?

- Good eating habits are essential for good health. Some specific foods and eating behaviors can affect pain levels. There is a lot of misinformation at present about nutritional therapies for pain.
- Studies of nutritional therapies are difficult to carry out for a number of reasons, and the results of such studies must be evaluated with extreme care.
- You can follow some basic nutritional recommendations now to improve your general health and help you in pain management.

Fresh Is Best; Moderation

- Foods prepared by others are more likely to have added salt, sugar, saturated fats, preservatives, and artificial color.

- Consuming a diet high in fat and sodium and low in fiber can put you at risk for developing heart disease, some cancers (colon), high blood pressure, and obesity.

- Eating fresh foods in moderation will help you maintain a stable weight that is appropriate for your height.

Basic Nutritional Guidelines

- The six basic food groups are:
    - —Grains (whole and refined)
    - —Vegetables
    - —Fruits
    - —Milk, yogurt, and cheese
    - —Meat, poultry, fish, dry beans, eggs, and nuts
    - —Oils
- Basic daily recommendations for healthy adults:
    - —Eat a variety of fruits, vegetables, whole grains, legumes (beans), fish, lean meat, and poultry.
    - —Each day eat five servings of vegetables and fruits and six servings of grain products (including whole grains). Eat two servings of a fatty fish per week.
    - —Use fat-free and low-fat dairy products.
- The six basic food groups provide us with our requirements of the following nutrients: carbohydrates, proteins, fats, and vitamins and minerals.

Managing Pain through Nutrition

- Keep a food diary (see sample at end of book) for several weeks to help you identify how, when, what, and why you eat. Look for any diet-associated patterns in your pain.

- Take the time to prepare yourself for eating. Try to eat without distractions, and pay attention to the nourishment you are taking into your body. After eating, take some time to sit quietly and let the food digest.

- Follow these "dos and don'ts" regarding when to eat:
    - —Do eat breakfast to get energy for your daily activities.
    - —Do not fast for prolonged periods, and avoid eating sweets as snacks.

—Don't skip meals.

—Don't eat most of your calories in the evening.

- Track what you eat and drink and whether it makes your pain condition better or worse. This tells you which foods to avoid and which foods to keep in your diet.

- Think about why you eat. This can help you see when you eat for psychological reasons (it's comforting, soothing) and when you need physical nourishment.

- Experiment with avoiding the following substances if you experience certain symptoms:

  —Caffeine (general pain, stress)

  —Alcohol (migraines or other headaches, general pain)

  —MSG (headaches, burning face, sweating, chest tightness)

  —Aspartame (headaches)

- At this time there is no consistent evidence that taking most vitamin or mineral supplements in addition to your normal diet is helpful in relieving pain. Calcium supplements need to be considered, however, because of the increased incidence of osteoporosis in postmenopausal women and older men that can lead to the bone fractures.

Exploration Tasks

1. Record everything you eat and drink for 1 week, using the food diary provided at the back of this book. At the end of the week, look over your diary and see where you might like to alter your diet.

   Or for 2 to 4 weeks eat a diet with no meat; lots of fruits, grains, and vegetables; no sweet snacks; and no alcohol or caffeine. If you are a big caffeine drinker, you may want to gradually decrease the amount of caffeine you drink so you won't suffer any withdrawal symptoms. Observe whether your pain is affected by the dietary change. If you sense any improvement, continue the diet for at least 2 months to give it a sufficient trial.

2. Set a goal that you want to accomplish related to your diet. Once again, make sure your goal is a behavioral task that you can measure in terms of the steps that *you* will take to accomplish it. Here is an example:

Goal: *Eat five servings of fruits and vegetables a day.*

Steps to take to reach that goal:

A. *List fruits and vegetables that I like.*

B. *Keep track of my intake of food and drink for a week.*

C. *Count up the number of servings of fruits and vegetables I eat a day.*

Now it's your turn.

Goal: _____

Steps to take to reach that goal:

A. _____

B. _____

C. _____

D. _____

In addition, list contingency plans. That is, identify what obstacles might get in the way of your accomplishing this goal. What solutions can you devise to work toward insuring the success of this goal?

	Obstacles	**Solutions**
A.	_____	_____
B.	_____	_____
C.	_____	_____
D.	_____	_____

3. Continue sharing your pleasurable activities. What kind of things have you enjoyed recently? _____

_____

4. What physical exercises have you been able to do on a regular basis? _____

_____

5. If some aspect of changing your nutritional habits (or any other facet of working with your pain) is causing you particular stress or anxiety, try imagining yourself in a safe, pleasant place (see Chapter 3, RR Technique 5). Describe your special place:

_____

_____

_____

Supplementary Reading

The following books and articles provide additional information on basic nutrition and on nutrition and pain. Also refer to the Internet Resources section at the back of the book for Web resources on nutrition.

American Heart Association, *American Heart Association Low-Fat, Low Cholesterol Cookbook, 3rd Edition: Delicious Recipes to Help Lower Your Cholesterol* (New York: Clarkson Potter, 2004).

L. Gail Darlington, "Dietary Therapy for Arthritis," *Rheumatic Disease Clinics of North America, 17*: 273–285, 1991.

Gail Darlington and Linda Gamlin, *Diet and Arthritis* (North Pomfret, VT: Trafalgar Square, 1998).

Johanna Dwyer, "Nutritional Remedies: Reasonable and Questionable," *Annals of Behavioral Medicine, 14*: 120–125, 1992.

Jens Kjeldsen-Kragh et al., "Controlled Trial of Fasting and One-Year Vegetarian Diet in Rheumatoid Arthritis," *Lancet, 338*: 899–902, 1991.

J. M. Kremer et al., "Effects of High Dose Fish Oil on Rheumatoid Arthritis after Stopping Nonsteroidal Anti-inflammatory Drugs: Clinical and Immune Correlates," *Arthritis and Rheumatology, 38*: 1107–1114, 1995.

Samara Joy Nielsen and Barry M. Popkin, "Patterns and Trends in Food Portion Sizes, 1977–1998," *Journal of the American Medical Association, 289*(4): 450–453, 2003.

D. C. Nordstrom et al., "Alpha Linoleic Acid in the Treatment of Rheumatoid Arthritis: A Double Blind, Placebo Controlled and Randomized Study: Flaxseed vs. Safflower Oil," *Rheumatology International, 14*: 231–234, 1995.

Nutrition Action Healthletter. For subscription information, write to the Center for Science in the Public Interest, P.O. Box 96611, Washington DC 20090-6611; e-mail *circ@cspinet.org*, or order online at *www.cspinet.org*.

Richard Panush, "Does Food Cause or Cure Arthritis?", *Rheumatic Disease Clinics of North America, 17*: 259–272, 1991.

Jean A. T. Pennington and Helen Nichols Church, *Bowes and Church's Food Values of Portions Commonly Used, Thirteenth Edition.* (New York: Harper & Row, 1980).

Portion Size. Research to Practice Series, No. 2 (Atlanta: Centers for Disease Control and Prevention, 2006). Available at *www.cdc.gov/nccdphp/dnpa/nutrition/pdf/portion_size_research.pdf*.

Cynthia Radnitz, "Food Triggered Migraine: A Critical Review," *Annals of Behavioral Medicine, 12*: 51–64, 1990.

Carol Ann Rinzler, *Nutrition for Dummies, Fourth Edition* (Hoboken, NJ: Wiley, 2006).

Tufts University Health & Nutrition Letter. P.O. Box 420235, Palm Coast, FL 32142. Available at *tuftshealthletter.com*.

Hope S. Warshaw and George Blackburn, *The Restaurant Companion: A Guide to Healthier Eating Out* (Chicago: Surrey Books, 1995).

Walter C. Willett and P. J. Skerrett, *Eat, Drink, and Be Healthy: The Harvard Medical School Guide to Healthy Eating* (New York: Free Press, 2005).

Andrew Weil, *Eating Well for Optimum Health: The Essential Guide to Food, Diet, and Nutrition* (New York: Knopf, 2000).

8
Effective Communication

If you loved me, you'd know what I mean.
—*Me, to my husband*

Communication skills enable you to get a message across, to express how you feel, to receive feedback, and to listen without judging. The reason a chapter on basic communication skills is included in a book on managing chronic pain is this: Pain patients feel much distress not only because of their pain but also because of trying to communicate with others about their pain.

There are three basic types of communication problems. Most people, with or without pain, experience these problems at some point:

1. There is a mismatch between the words people speak (their statements) and what they really want (their intentions).

2. People do not state clearly how they feel, what they want, or what they need (assertiveness). They tend either to deny their own feelings ("You count, I don't"—passiveness) or to disregard the feelings of others ("I count, you don't"—aggressiveness).

3. People hear, but they don't really *listen* (active listening).

This chapter describes all three types of problems and provides suggestions for overcoming them.

Making Statements Match Intentions

General Communication: A Sample Scenario

Let's take a look at the following scenario:

You just came back from shopping, having bought a dress for slightly more money than you would normally spend. This was a treat for participating in the pain program, so you feel only slightly guilty. You put the dress on for dinner that night.

When your husband comes home, you ignore at first his observation that the trash barrels have not been brought in. Finally you say, "Well, what do you think?" (You realize that this is a loaded question, given the expense of the dress.)

"About the trash barrels?" he says, only slightly bewildered.

"The dress, the dress!" you exclaim.

"It's okay," he mumbles, really confused now.

You storm out of the room screaming about how insensitive and self-centered he is. You feel that if he loved you, he would know what you mean and want. He is thoroughly baffled.

The first principle of effective communication is to be clear about what you really want to say to others. (I confess I act at times as if my spouse is a mind reader, but doing this really does not help communication with him or anyone else.) Matching statements with intentions is an art and a skill. It also requires you to be responsible for your side of the conversation.

Let's go back to the scenario you just read. If your intention is to get feedback that you deserve this dress and you look great in it, then you could play Twenty Questions. Or you could say something like this: "I bought myself a dress today as a 'pick-me-up.' I'm looking for confirmation that I deserve to treat myself to this, and that you think I look great."

Some people feel that "it doesn't count" unless praise comes spontaneously from the other person. Although the other person (for example, the husband in the scenario above) does not have to respond in the way you wish, what you ask will be a lot clearer if your statement reflects your intent. He or she is still left with the option to comply or not.

Communication with Health Care Professionals: Put It in Writing

The following practice exercise may be useful for interactions with health care professionals, which can often be confusing and frustrating because of the mismatch of statements and intentions. Do not read further until you've done this exercise.

1. Assume that your pain has become worse. You go to the doctor. What do you say? Write out a statement to your physician. (It is important that you make this an *imaginary* interaction, not one that has actually occurred between you and your physician.)

_____

_____

_____

_____

2. Now, write what you want the doctor to say back to you.

_____

_____

_____

_____

In many of our interactions with others, we wish to receive the following:

- Information
- Analysis
- Advice
- Understanding
- Reassurance

If you have completed the exercise above, you can see what you wanted by looking at the doctor's statement to you. Were you asking for information, advice, analysis, reassurance, understanding, or some combination of these?

If you are like most people, your imaginary statement to the doctor was something like this: "My pain is worse—I hurt more now than ever." End of sentence! If you want advice, analysis, or reassurance, then you'll be disappointed in real life if the doctor says, "It's nothing. Take two aspirin and call me in the morning."

Try rewriting your first statement to your doctor. This time, however, include clear requests for advice, analysis, information, understanding, and/or reassurance. Here is an example: "My pain is worse. I would like you to examine me and run the appropriate tests to see if this is just a flare-up or something new. Should I change anything in terms of treatment? I'm scared, so I would appreciate it if you would do this to reassure me."

_____

_____

_____

_____

A lot of people find that asking for advice, analysis, or information is easy compared with asking for understanding or reassurance. Sometimes it's because they expect the latter to be automatic: "If you cared about me, you'd know what I want." It may also have to do with feeling that they are undeserving of this kind of attention or respect.

Doing this exercise can also uncover a "secret" desire for a cure or a miracle. If you are looking for miracles, be up front about it and ask directly. Then you and your physician can at least discuss the newest treatments or lack of them.

Deborah Tannen, author of *You Just Don't Understand* (see "Supplementary Reading"), says that giving advice is a common male communication response. If this is correct, then it may explain why many women patients complain that they do not get statements of reassurance or understanding from the predominantly male medical profession. In fact, women may not even think to ask for such statements. Many medical doctors simply do not feel that statements of reassurance and understanding are relevant in standard exchanges; others feel that they demonstrate understanding or reassurance by giving advice or sharing information.

Clearly, if you do not feel the need for reassurance, understanding, or any other item on the list above, then you do not need to ask for it. You are seeking clarification of your unique agenda. If your intentions are unclear or indirectly stated, you will not get what you need. You will feel misunderstood, used, and abused. Of course, just making it clear what you want does not guarantee that you will get it. But I believe you will be pleasantly surprised at the results once you begin practicing clearer communication.

Here are other suggestions for improving your interactions with health care professionals. They can help you prepare for your next doctor visit, no matter what symptoms you have. So before your next visit, do the following:

1. Write down your questions, listing the most important ones first.

2. Be ready to describe the symptom or problem that has brought you to the doctor. Keep the description simple and brief.

3. Ask yourself these questions about your symptoms or problem:

    Where is it located?

    When did it start? When does it occur?

    Describe the sensation (symptom): Is it sharp, burning, throbbing, aching, or the like?

    What makes it better?

    What makes it worse?

    What have you done about it?

4. If the problem is related to your chronic pain, it is important to be very specific about your symptoms. Ask yourself:

Is the pain more severe? How so?

Has the pain quality changed (for example, it was tingling, now it's burning)?

Has the location of your pain changed (for example, it was in your lower back and now it's down the back of your right leg)?

Are you experiencing additional symptoms (for example, spasm, fever, loss of bladder or bowel control, weight loss) with your pain?

Write down your answers to these questions and bring them with you. Many diagnoses are made from the patterns and interactions of symptoms, so this is important information. You may find it helpful to bring a chart of your pain levels (or symptom patterns).

5. Know what medications you are taking and the dosage for each. Bring the medication list you completed for Chapter 2 with you. Don't forget to include over-the-counter medications, herbals, and other supplements you're taking.

6. If you feel that there is a particular issue you need to discuss in detail that requires more than a 15-minute appointment, state this when you call your health care professional. The receptionist is not a mind reader, either.

7. Clarify your expectations. During your visit, are you looking for a miracle, a diagnosis, a treatment plan, or a prognosis?

The Weekly Feedback Sheet provided at the end of this book can also help you communicate clearly and explicitly with health care professionals.

After listening to your history and doing an examination related to your symptoms, the health care professional should be able to give you an opinion on what is going on or what might be investigated further. He or she should then give you a plan that may include diagnostic tests, medication or changes in medication, other non-drug therapies, and education. Ask for this in writing if you think you will not remember what is being said or do not have a family member with you.

If you are given a new medication or therapy, track your symptom in your pain diary over the next week or more (depending on treatment). Have the symptoms that brought you to the office changed? How have they changed and when did they change? This will be important feedback for your clinician. Often therapies and medications are started but then there is little discussion of whether they make enough of a difference to warrant continued use. As a result, people continue injection therapies, physical therapy, or medication long after their effectiveness is past.

Assertiveness

"Assertiveness" means expressing how you feel while respecting the rights of others: "I count, you count." There are three common obstacles to becoming assertive:

1. You do not feel entitled to speak up about how you feel, what you want, or what you need.

2. You confuse assertiveness with passiveness ("You count, I don't") or with aggression ("I count, you don't").

3. You don't know why you feel the way you do, either because you never thought about it or because you are communicating in a style that is based on past assumptions or attitudes.

Obstacle 1: Not Feeling Entitled to Speak Up

Just as you learn irrational beliefs and cognitive distortions, you learn certain "rules" of communication early in life:

"It's not proper to speak unless spoken to."

"Children should be seen and not heard."

"You have to answer all inquiries. If questioned, you can't say 'I don't know.' "

"You should always accommodate others. It's not right to say no."

From these subtle rules, you learn to suppress your opinion. According to Deborah Tannen (see "Supplementary Reading"), you have learned this thoroughly if you are a woman. Women receive different messages about communicating than men do, and one of these is that women should not speak up for themselves.

Many of you may still feel uncomfortable about speaking up for what you feel, want, or need. You may find it helpful to consider assertiveness as a two-way street. You do have a right to express your opinion about how you feel and what you want or think you need; however, there are responsibilities that go along with those rights, which involve your awareness of the rights, wants, and needs of others. Melodie Chenevert, a nurse, writes about the need for rights and responsibilities in her book *Special Techniques in Assertiveness Training*:

Rights–Responsibilities

Rights	Responsibilities
To speak up	To listen
To take	To give
To have problems	To find solutions
To be comforted	To comfort others
To work	To do your best
To make mistakes	To correct your mistakes
To laugh	To make others happy

(cont.)

Rights	Responsibilities
To have friends	To be a friend
To criticize	To praise
To have your efforts rewarded	To reward others' efforts
To independence	To be dependable
To cry	To dry tears
To be loved	To love others

From Melodie Chenevert, *Special Techniques in Assertiveness Training: STAT* (St. Louis: C. V. Mosby, 1988, p. 64). Copyright 1988 by C. V. Mosby. Reprinted by permission.

Take time to add other rights and responsibilities to those listed here. The assertive person knows that abusing either rights or responsibilities is self-destructive.

Obstacle 2: Confusing Assertiveness with Passiveness or Aggression

Let's consider three basic styles of interpersonal behavior—passive, aggressive, and assertive—from the perspective of our previous discussion. What are the intentions of passive, aggressive, and assertive statements?

Statement	Intention
Passive	
"Okay, whatever you say, I don't care." "Do whatever you want to do [sigh]."	To keep the peace, I don't make waves; I compromise even when it is not called for. You count, I don't.
Aggressive	
"You are a jerk! It's all your fault." "I don't care what you say." "You'll do what I say."	To win, I punish, blame, or strike back whenever I think it is necessary. I count, you don't.
Assertive	
"I feel sad when you don't ask what I would like to do, because it makes me think you don't care about me or about what I would like. I want you to ask me what I would like to do. I will promise to come up with some ideas or not hold you responsible if I don't."	I express my feelings, define the behavior that gives rise to those feelings, and state the reason I feel the way I do. Adding "I want" and "I will" expands the assertive statement by describing a desired action and identifying my responsibility in this interaction. I count, you count.

The advantage of speaking assertively is that it gives you the opportunity to express your point of view. However, this style also demands a certain honesty about, and a clear understanding of, what it is you really want. Hence, we have the third obstacle to assertiveness.

Obstacle 3: Not Knowing Why You Feel the Way You Do

What do you want? Why do you want it?

The "formula" for assertive communication is as follows:

"I feel _____ when you _____ because _____."

This formula requires that *all three* elements be included. Many people get stuck after "I feel"; completing the rest of the sentence means getting in touch with yourself and exploring your inner feelings. Let's take a look at why it's important to do so.

For almost 2 years Paul had suffered a painful diabetic neuropathy involving his hands and lower extremities. He had become unable to do his job as a plumber. Out of work for 6 months, he found himself bored and irritable.

One day his oldest child came home from school and made the comment that it was cold in the house. Paul became enraged and stormed out to the garage, where he commonly retreated when he became upset. He said to himself, "It didn't feel cold to me, the child must be a wimp." Upon further reflection, however, he found himself making statements like "It's the father's responsibility to provide warmth, food, and protection to his family. If I can't provide for my family, then I'm worthless."

Paul had not been aware of how distressed he was about not being able to work. He went back into the house, and after dinner discussed his feelings with his family. His oldest child informed him that the pilot light had gone out on the gas furnace and that he had relit it. They all had a good laugh when Paul told them how angry he had felt when his son commented about the heat, and how he had taken it as a sign that he couldn't even provide his family with the basics, such as warmth.

Once Paul was able to express his concerns in an assertive way, he was able to receive the reassurance from his family that they understood and did not think him any less of a father or provider because he was not working outside the home.

Theresa, another patient, expressed frustration over a bathroom remodeling project that was going on at home. She found herself extremely irritated with her husband when he showed her a set of faucets that he thought might look nice in the bathroom. She was outraged and responded that the faucets would be hard to clean and that she was the one who would be cleaning them.

When Theresa was asked to turn her response into an assertive statement to

---

her husband, she said, "I feel annoyed when you show me fancy faucets to put in the bathroom because for the past 25 years you have never taken what I do into consideration. You always take me for granted." She was deluged with and surprised by feelings resulting from 25 years of marital frustrations. An important thing to keep in mind about assertive messages is that they cannot be used to correct all past damages and unspoken hurts. Theresa was able to see this and realized that her responsibility was to decide what she really wanted to communicate. She also realized that she and her husband needed to do much more talking and be less silent with each other.

Theresa's statements then became this: "I feel conflicted when you ask for my approval of fancy faucets because, while they are very pretty, I would find them hard to clean. When you present me with what seem to be thoughtless choices, I wonder if you ever think about all that I do at home when you're at work." Actually, as it turned out, her husband had never thought of it that way. He was able to appreciate why she might not be ecstatic about his choice of faucets, and Theresa was able to feel proud that she had stood up for herself.

"I want" statements help direct the action you want. When there is a need for compromise or clarification, "I will" statements help the other person agree to your request. For example, Theresa might have said to her husband, "If you bring me a catalogue of faucets, I will make an effort to choose one that suits my needs."

It's important to differentiate between a hurtful and aggressive statement and one that is used to clarify your feelings or intentions. For example, the statement "I feel you are a jerk" is not assertive, even though it begins with "I feel." Although aggressive statements may flow more easily than assertive ones, they rarely accomplish anything except revenge ("I showed them"), which is usually short-lived. They complicate further communication or eliminate it altogether.

Passive statements, such as "It's up to you" or "I don't care," may be appropriate at times when used judiciously and consciously. If they merely reinforce martyrdom or self-abuse, then they too will poison communication and relationships.

The major difficulties in beginning assertive communication are (1) becoming conscious of why you feel the way you do and (2) taking responsibility for how you feel, rather than blaming others or wishing things could be different. One of the reasons that Chapter 5 gives you the opportunity to identify negative self-talk and other negative responses is to help you overcome these difficulties. Although at first it may seem uncomfortable or awkward to state directly how you feel, it allows true dialogue (two-way communication). Completing the Assertiveness Questionnaire, provided at the end of this chapter, will help you identify situations in which assertiveness may be awkward for you.

Active Listening

Active listening is a technique that can de-escalate (or at least clarify) many emotional exchanges. It is a first step in conflict resolution and prevention. Active listening requires truly hearing what someone else is saying—*not* judging, parroting, questioning, supporting, rationalizing, or defending.

For example, suppose that your spouse announces, "I'm fed up with how the house always looks." Now this is understandably a loaded statement, because you may already be feeling uneasy about your inability to keep up with things when you have a pain problem. Here are some unhelpful replies:

- *Judging*: "You shouldn't feel that way."

- *Parroting*: "So you don't like the way the house looks?"

- *Questioning*: "Really? Do you have any brilliant ideas on how to keep up with it?"

- *Supporting*: "Things will get better. I'll try harder."

- *Rationalizing*: "You've had a hard day at work. Sit down and cool off."

- *Defending*: "I do the best I can, but you're never satisfied."

Some of these statements sound more reasonable than others, but each one ends the discussion prematurely—either by jumping to conclusions, not allowing further information, or putting off conversation.

A phrase that can be useful in these cases comes from the work of psychologist Carl Rogers:

"You sound _____ about _____."

Let's fill in the blanks to explore the above scenario further: "You sound *upset* about *not keeping the house up*." Possible responses from your spouse include the following:

"Oh, it's not just here; it's the chaos at work. I feel so overwhelmed because I can't get things done. I have two projects due. . . ."

"You better believe I'm upset. I work hard all day and I don't like coming home to a house in disarray."

With active listening, you buy time and get a better idea of what the other person is feeling. Then you can make a choice between expending the energy or effort to answer, or deciding not to involve yourself in the other person's distress. Once you have decided to reply, it can be very rewarding to deflect responses that are potential sources of conflict. You can do this by first acknowledging how the other person feels; this permits both parties to respect their differences. Second, clarify the actual source of distress. This second step eases discussion onto neutral ground where problem solving can occur. For example, "You better believe I'm upset . . ."

might be followed by this: "I'm sorry you're upset. I wanted to check out whether it was me, the way the house looks, or something else that was bothering you." From here, the conversation could proceed to problem solving—that is, how to handle the fact that the house is in disarray and that it may be difficult to keep up with maintaining it.

Active listening thus serves to defuse emotional energies that can quickly escalate into confrontation. It also allows you to be reflective, empathic, objective, and nonjudgmental. By naming the other person's feelings you encourage him or her to further express them. By clarifying what these feelings are about, you promote problem solving and reinforce a healthier expression of emotions. Like any new behavior, active listening takes practice—but it is well worth the effort.

Further Suggestions for Communication Practice

People have a difficult time changing their communication styles. Perhaps this is because they think little about communication once they have learned to speak. Some suggestions, however, may help you practice. In the beginning, as with monitoring your self-talk, the process can appear long and laborious. But the more you practice, the easier it will get. Notice when you experience interpersonal conflict or discomfort. This is a good time to pause and reflect on where the communication problem might be. Has your intent been clearly stated? Are you being passive or aggressive out of habit? Have you considered where the other person is coming from, or have you simply assumed you know? Is it a gender-based or cultural conflict that involves communication styles, not personality issues?

An experience I had on a trip with a group of Spanish, English, and American tourists illustrates the last of these points. We stopped in a small Greek resort town to eat lunch. After we had waited in the buffet line for over an hour, the problem became apparent. We overheard various English and Spanish groups discussing it with great animation. Each nationality was accusing the other of "queuing up" (that is, lining up) from the "wrong" side. The English claimed that "everyone knows you queue from the left"; the Spanish were just as vehement about queuing from the right. (The Americans, of course, just barged right into the middle of the line.) The conflict, which quickly became personalized, was based on cultural factors that no group was willing or able to acknowledge at the time. Major battles have probably been started over misunderstandings of even lesser magnitude and significance.

Taking responsibility for our words and thoughts is not easy. We tend automatically to apply long-held, often unexamined, attitudes to our problems. Our solutions are too often quick fixes that may not hold up over the longer term. Communication habits are hard to change but few of us can afford to indulge in ways of thinking that don't really work. As you will see for yourself, practicing effective communication skills can make your life a great deal easier.

Summary

- There are three important aspects of communication: making statements match intentions, assertiveness, and active listening.

- Making statements match intentions refers to saying clearly what you really want. This is particularly important in communication with health care providers. Make it plain what you are requesting: information, analysis, advice, understanding, and/or reassurance.

- Assertiveness is a positive and direct way of expressing how you feel while respecting the rights of others. There are three common obstacles to becoming assertive:

    —Not feeling entitled to speak up

    —Confusing assertiveness with passiveness or aggression

    —Not knowing why you feel the way you do

- The formula for assertive statements is: "I feel _____ when you _____ because _____."

- Active listening is a conscious technique; it requires truly hearing what someone else is saying without assuming that you know what the person is trying to say.

- After active listening, a useful response that can de-escalate or clarify emotional exchanges is to say "You sound _____ about _____."

Exploration Tasks

1. Complete the Assertiveness Questionnaire, provided at the end of this chapter. What did you learn?

_____

_____

_____

How might you more effectively manage those situations in which assertiveness is a problem for you?

_____

_____

_____

_____

2. Identify an assertive communication: As you go through your week, be aware of any difficult conversations—situations in which you either spoke assertively or did not but should have. Write down the key elements of the dialogue in one conversation.

I said: _____

_____

_____

The other person said: _____

_____

_____

I said: _____

_____

_____

He or she said: _____

_____

_____

I said: _____

_____

_____

Once you have recorded the conversation, analyze it in terms of the assertive communication guidelines discussed in this chapter. Did you use "I" sentences ("I feel," "I want," etc.)? Did you describe the specific behavior that was troubling you and why? Did you express your opinion and views and respect those of the other person? Finally, look at what followed the conversation. If you were assertive, what stress do you think you avoided? If you were not assertive, what stress did you create for yourself?

3. Continue to keep track of your negative self-talk and other negative responses, using the worksheet provided at the end of the book for this purpose. Now, consider this question: How can you reframe those thoughts to reflect the reality of the situation, using "I can" and "I need" statements? Pay particular attention to those situations involving conflict in communication with others. What is the source of the conflict as you see it? Are there unspoken assumptions or expectations involved? Do you have the "whole picture," or do you need more information?

4. Practice the "You sound _____ about _____" listening response to the following statements, and then use an assertive response ("I feel _____ when you _____ because _____") to practice stating your intent. Use the "I want" and "I will" statements, too.

A. "You should be better by now! There is nothing wrong on X-rays or blood tests, and yet you still have pain. I have nothing more to offer you!"

Listening response: _____

_____

_____

Assertive response: _____

_____

_____

B. "Every time I call you to do something, you give me this vague story about not knowing if you'll be able to go."

Listening response: _____

_____

_____

Assertive response: _____

_____

_____

C. "What is this, a perpetual vacation? When are you going back to work, or don't you want to give up a good thing?"

Listening response: _____

_____

_____

Assertive response: _____

_____

_____

5. Write out a goal that you want to accomplish related to the material in this chapter. As always, make sure your goal is a behavioral task that you can measure in terms of the steps *you* will take to accomplish it. Here is an example:

Goal: To practice clear communication with my doctor at my next visit.

Steps to take to reach that goal:

A. Clarify my expectations of the visit by writing out a statement to the doctor. Make sure it reflects my intentions.

B. Chart my pain on a graph so that the preceding four-week pattern is displayed.

C. Bring my medication list with me.

D. Write out my questions before I go, putting the most important ones first.

Now it's your turn.

Goal: _____

Steps to take to reach that goal:

A. _____

B. _____

C. _____

D. _____

In addition, list contingency plans. That is, identify what obstacles might get in the way of your accomplishing this goal. What solutions can you devise to work toward insuring the success of this goal?

Obstacles	**Solutions**
A. _____	_____
B. _____	_____
C. _____	_____
D. _____	_____

6. Now is a good time to start exploring RR Technique 7 (see Chapter 3), if you have not already tried it. After you have worked with the pain image, you can put other problems behind the clear plastic wall to examine. Distancing yourself from a problem this way can help you develop an objective view of the issue and perhaps become more effective at problem solving.

Supplementary Reading

The following books provide additional information on communication skills:

David Burns, *The Feeling Good Handbook* (New York: Plume, 1999).

David Burns, *Ten Days to Self-Esteem* (New York: Quill/William Morrow, 1999).

Martha Davis, Matthew McKay, and Elizabeth Robbins Eshelman, *The Relaxation and Stress Reduction Workbook* (Oakland, CA: New Harbinger, 2000).

Roger Fisher and William Ury, *Getting to Yes: Negotiating Agreement without Giving In* (New York: Penguin, 1991).

Marshall Rosenberg and Arun Gandhi, *Nonviolent Communication: A Language of Life* (Encinitas, CA: PuddleDancer Press, 2005).

Larry A. Samovar, Richard E. Porter, and Edwin R. McDaniel, *Communication between Cultures* (Wadsworth Series in Communication Studies) (Boston, MA: Thomson Learning, 2006).

Jenny Steinmetz, Jon Blankenship, Linda Brown, Deborah Hall, and Grace Miller, *Managing Stress Before It Manages You* (Palo Alto, CA: Bull, 1980).

Deborah Tannen, *The Power of Talk: Who Gets Heard and Why (HBR OnPoint Enhanced Edition),* e-document download available through Amazon.com, January 5, 2008.

Deborah Tannen, *That's Not What I Meant! How Conversational Style Makes or Breaks Relationships* (New York: Ballantine Books, 1992).

Deborah Tannen, *You Just Don't Understand: Women and Men in Conversation* (New York: Harper Paperbacks, 2001).

Assertiveness Questionnaire

To further refine your assessment of the situations in which you need to be more assertive, complete the following questionnaire. Put a check mark in column A by the items that are applicable to you and then rate those items in column B as:

    1. Comfortable
    2. Mildly uncomfortable
    3. Moderately uncomfortable
    4. Very uncomfortable
    5. Unbearably threatening

(Note that the varying degrees of discomfort can be expressed whether your inappropriate reactions are hostile or passive.)

A	B	
Check here if the item applies to you	Rate from 1–5 for discomfort	*When* do you behave nonassertively?
_____	_____	Asking for help
_____	_____	Stating a difference of opinion
_____	_____	Receiving and expressing negative feelings
_____	_____	Receiving and expressing positive feelings
_____	_____	Dealing with someone who refuses to cooperate
_____	_____	Speaking up about something that annoys you
_____	_____	Talking when all eyes are on you
_____	_____	Protesting a rip-off
_____	_____	Saying "No"
_____	_____	Responding to undeserved criticism
_____	_____	Making requests of authority figures
_____	_____	Negotiating for something you want
_____	_____	Having to take charge
_____	_____	Asking for cooperation
_____	_____	Proposing an idea
_____	_____	Taking charge
_____	_____	Asking questions

(cont.)

From Martha Davis, Elizabeth Robbins Eshelman, and Matthew McKay, *The Relaxation and Stress Reduction Workbook* (Oakland, CA: New Harbinger, 1988). Copyright 1988 by New Harbinger Publications. Reprinted by permission.

Assertiveness Questionnaire *(cont.)*

A	**B**	
Check here if the item applies to you	Rate from 1–5 for discomfort	*When* do you behave nonassertively?
_____	_____	Dealing with attempts to make you feel guilty
_____	_____	Asking for service
_____	_____	Asking for a date or appointment
_____	_____	Asking for favors
_____	_____	Other: _____

A	**B**	
Check here if the item applies to you	Rate from 1–5 for discomfort	*Who* are the people with whom you are nonassertive?
_____	_____	Parents
_____	_____	Fellow workers or classmates
_____	_____	Strangers
_____	_____	Old friends
_____	_____	Spouse or mate
_____	_____	Employer
_____	_____	Relatives
_____	_____	Children
_____	_____	Acquaintances
_____	_____	Salespeople, clerks, hired help
_____	_____	More than two or three people in a group
_____	_____	Other: _____

A	**B**	
Check here if the item applies to you	Rate from 1–5 for discomfort	*What* do you want that you have been unable to achieve with nonassertive styles?
_____	_____	Approval for things that you have done well
_____	_____	To get help with certain tasks
_____	_____	More attention or time with your mate
_____	_____	To be listened to and understood
_____	_____	To make boring or frustrating situations more satisfying

_____	_____	To not have to be nice all the time
_____	_____	Confidence in speaking up when something is important to you
_____	_____	Greater comfort with strangers, store clerks, mechanics, etc.
_____	_____	Confidence in asking for contact with people you find attractive
_____	_____	To get a new job, ask for interviews, raises, and so on
_____	_____	Comfort with people who supervise you or work under you
_____	_____	To not feel angry and bitter a lot of the time
_____	_____	To overcome a feeling of helplessness and the sense that nothing ever really changes
_____	_____	To initiate satisfying sexual experiences
_____	_____	To do something totally different and novel
_____	_____	To have time by yourself
_____	_____	To do things that are fun or relaxing for you
_____	_____	Other: _____

Evaluating Your Responses

Examine your answers for an overall picture of what situations and people you find most threatening. How does nonassertive behavior keep you from attaining the specific items you checked on the "What" list? In putting together your own assertiveness program, focus first on items you rated as falling in the 2–3 range. These are the situations that you will find easiest to change. Items that are very uncomfortable or threatening can be tackled later.

9
Effective Problem Solving

The problems that exist in the world cannot be solved by the level of thinking that created them.

—*Albert Einstein*

People often get caught up in trying to solve problems before they are prepared to do so. In reading earlier chapters, you may have thought problem solving was the next logical step. But to be prepared, you first need to be able to quiet your mind chatter through RR techniques. You need to clarify what you think and feel, and understand how your attitudes can affect your ability to cope with stress. You need to know your communication style and improve your communication skills. To solve problems effectively you need to set clear goals, identify emotional barriers (hooks), and come up with a sequence of small steps needed to reach the goal. Now you are ready to begin problem solving.

Setting Goals: A Closer Look

Take a moment to write down three goals that you would like to accomplish in the next 6 months. You have been asked to set goals at the end of each chapter, so the task has probably become less difficult. If you need to refresh your memory on setting goals, refer to Chapter 1.

1. Goal: _____

2. Goal: _____

3. Goal: _____

As you may have discovered, accomplishing goals can be much more difficult than setting them. Failing to reach your goals often has little or nothing to do with the smaller steps you've planned. For example, let's take a look at a goal set by Barbara, a patient with pain.

The Emotional Hook

One of Barbara's goals was to go back to work. I asked her why she hadn't done it before this. After mentioning her pain and saying she didn't know what to do, she suddenly paused. "You know, the truth is . . . I'm terrified at the prospect." I asked her to write about the problem—her terror—in the format used to examine the automatic thoughts or self-talk associated with negative emotions:

Situation	Thought	Emotion	Distortion
Going back to work	"I'll never keep up"	Terrified	Jumping to conclusions
	"I'll reinjure myself"	Anxious	Fortune telling

What Barbara was experiencing can be called an "emotional hook." Picture those long vaudeville hooks that pulled bad acts off the stage. Emotional hooks are the cognitive distortions explored in Chapter 5. They are the source of self-defeating talk and they block your ability to solve problems.

As long as Barbara remained terrified about whether she could perform at work or might be reinjured, her emotional hook would pull her away (like a bad vaudeville act) from her goal (and her show would not go on!). Emotional hooks need to be dealt with before real problem solving can begin. Fortunately, you already have the tools to cope with emotional hooks; they are the same ones you use to deal with negative self-talk. First, identify your feelings, your self-talk, and the cognitive distortions and irrational beliefs behind them. Then challenge the reality of those thoughts.

Barbara challenged the thoughts behind her fear. According to objective tests administered by her occupational health specialist, her pain problem was chronic and a regular work routine was not going to harm her. She knew that she could ask for reasonable accommodations in the workplace if she was partially disabled or impaired under the Americans with Disabilities Act (see "Supplementary Reading"). She had been practicing alternating pain-increasing activities with pain-decreasing activities for a while. She would adjust this to her work routine using the sticky note ideas from Chapter 4. She knew that she would need to continue her exercise program, communicate her need to change positions throughout her workday, and regularly destress herself with mini-relaxations. She was now ready to feel the fear but do it anyway!

Identifying the Barriers to Accomplishing Your Goals

> That which we do not bring to consciousness appears in our life as fate.
>
> —*Carl Gustav Jung*

Can you identify an emotional hook keeping you from accomplishing one of your goals? Start by asking why you haven't achieved your goal yet or else pick a goal you feel will be difficult to achieve. (The goals you think are difficult often harbor emotional hooks.) When you consider this goal, are you aware of feeling anxious, fearful, or overwhelmed? Identify the emotion you feel, then put it in the same format that Barbara did above: identify the self-talk (the hook) and the cognitive distortions that go with it. How will you challenge your thoughts? After you've done that, look again at your goal. Now, what is the "problem" that needs solving? Solving the actual problem is often surprisingly easy, once it is untangled from the emotional hook.

Here's an exercise in identifying an emotional hook and then restating the problem:

Write down one of your goals that feels difficult. (Check the goals you wrote at the beginning of this chapter.)

Goal: _____

When you think about why you haven't accomplished this goal up to now or why you think it might be difficult, what do you feel? For example: overwhelmed, anxious, fearful.

Feelings (emotional response): _____

What kind of self-talk do you find yourself doing when you think about this emotion or the difficulty of the goal? For example, "I can't do it. What if I fail?"

Self-talk (automatic thoughts) (a.k.a. emotional hook): _____

_____

Next, identify the source of the self-talk in terms of distortions, catastrophizing, avoidance, denial, and irrational beliefs. For example, "I shouldn't have to make changes, it wasn't my fault" = cognitive distortion; "Life should be fair" = irrational belief; "This is the worst thing that could happen and I can't take it" = catastrophizing.

Cognitive distortion or irrational beliefs (Chapter 5)/**Negative attitudes** (Chapter 6):

_____

_____

Now challenge the thoughts that are unrealistic and reflect on the reality of the situation you find yourself in. What can you do and what do you need? If you get stuck, use the vertical arrow technique (see Chapter 5) or write about your problem for 20 minutes and see what comes up. For example: "It's not fair that I have to change how I do things, but this is about going forward, creating a new life with pain. What is required is my changing how I do things."

Challenges to self-talk: _____

_____

_____

How do you feel now about the possibility of accomplishing your goal? Relieved, sad, but committed?

Now you are in a better position to plan the steps for achieving your goal because, having faced the source of your goblins and ghouls, you won't let them sabotage your success!

Identifying the Steps Needed for Goal Achievement

When planning how to reach your goal, it is important to break it down into many small steps, particularly if it is an ambitious goal. These small steps can be grouped into smaller goals. This will help to guarantee your successful accomplishment of the larger goal.

For example, Barbara's goal was to return to work. She broke that large goal down into the following smaller steps: She would update her résumé, determine what kind of job she wanted and could do, get help from the state's vocational rehabilitation services, and start getting job applications. She would continue to do her exercise routine but split it up between the morning and afternoon or evening to accommodate a work schedule. She would make sure that she had a routine of getting up and going to bed at the same time. She identified friends that she could talk with should she begin to feel overwhelmed and made a commitment to continue attending church weekly to get the spiritual support she needed. She moved her relaxation technique to bedtime to make sure she would go to sleep in the most relaxed state. She identified some cookbooks that could assist her in cooking quick but healthy meals. She checked with her occupational therapist to review assistive devices that she might incorporate into her work performance. Barbara could now move toward accomplishing her return to work.

Note that the steps for Barbara's goal of succeeding in her return to work could be spelled out and subdivided further. The more you define the steps, the more likely you are to accomplish the goal.

Contingency plans are also helpful. I first described those in the "Exploration Tasks" for Chapter 3. These plans keep you from failing. For example, if Barbara's pain was getting worse away from home, she made plans for a private place she could go to elicit the RR. She also arranged for a massage therapist to call if her pain flared up.

Take your goal and break it down into the steps you will need to take to reach it. Be as specific as you can, dividing each step into smaller steps whenever necessary.

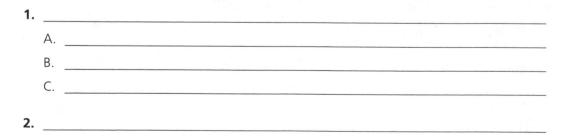

1. _____

    A. _____

    B. _____

    C. _____

2. _____

A. _____

B. _____

C. _____

3. _____

A. _____

B. _____

C. _____

4. _____

A. _____

B. _____

C. _____

Now list contingency plans. As in earlier chapters' "Exploration Tasks," remember to define these in terms of possible obstacles and their solutions.

Obstacles	**Solutions**
_____	_____
_____	_____
_____	_____
_____	_____

Assessing Your Ways of Coping and Applying Them to Problems

If you started at the beginning of this book and did all the exercises, you now have many coping skills. To help remember what you've learned, think of the skills as grouped in the following way:

- Physical ways of coping
- Emotion-focused coping
- Problem-focused coping

The physical ways of coping include aerobic exercise, labeling your sensations, pacing your activities, RR techniques, and so on. The emotion-focused coping skills include RR techniques, capturing negative self-talk and challenging it, assertiveness, and so forth. The problem-focused coping skills include setting goals, seeking pleasurable activities, identifying resources for obtaining more information, brainstorming with friends and associates, securing social support, and the like.

You will note that a particular skill may fall into more than one category, depending on how it is used and for what purpose. For example, an RR technique can be used to calm a tense body (physical coping), as well as a tense emotional state (emotion-focused coping).

When people ask friends or relatives for help in solving problems, there is often an immediate move to problem solving: "Have you tried this or that?" or "My aunt had that problem and she did this." As you have seen earlier in this chapter, moving to problem solving too early and too quickly can doom it if there is an emotional hook. Such hooks require you to cope with the emotion component. Similarly, people who have used only physical ways of coping (for example, strenuous exercise) for stress management can become very depressed when chronic pain reduces physical activity. You need to have a variety of coping skills and know when to use them to manage life problems in general and chronic pain in particular.

This program offers a variety of skills. You have probably gravitated to some skills more than others and found some skills more difficult than others. But keep practicing all of them.

Take some time to go back through the book to see whether you can identify all the skills you have learned. Can you organize the skills into the three categories below? Put an asterisk (*) by the ones you still need to work on. Creating a list of your skills will come in handy when we discuss planning for pain flare-ups.

Physical ways of coping: _____

_____

_____

_____

_____

_____

Emotion-focused coping skills: _____

_____

_____

_____

_____

_____

Problem-focused coping skills: _____

_____

_____

_____

_____

_____

The following poem (from Portia Nelson's *There's a Hole in My Sidewalk*; see Bibliography) summarizes the self-discovery process—the same process you have begun by reading this book.

An Autobiography in Five Chapters

Chapter 1
    I walk down the street.
    There is a deep hole in the sidewalk. I fall in.
    I am lost. . . . I am helpless. It isn't my fault.
    It takes forever to find a way out.

Chapter 2
    I walk down the same street.
    There is a deep hole in the sidewalk.
    I pretend I don't see it.
    I fall in again.
    I can't believe I am in this same place.
    But it isn't my fault.
    It still takes a long time to get out.

Chapter 3
    I walk down the same street.
    There is a deep hole in the sidewalk.
    I see it is there.
    I fall in . . . it's a habit . . . but my eyes are open.
    I know where I am.
    It is my fault.
    I get out immediately.

Chapter 4
    I walk down the same street.
    There is a deep hole in the sidewalk.
    I walk around it.

Chapter 5
    I walk down a different street.

                           —*Portia Nelson*

Summary

- If you find a goal difficult to accomplish, do the following:
  - —Look for an emotional hook (negative automatic thoughts or self-defeating talk).
  - —Identify the emotional hook and the cognitive distortions that go with it.
  - —Challenge and change the self-talk.
  - —Now restate the goal.
- Identify the smaller steps you need to take to solve a problem or reach a goal; the more you break down and define the steps, the more likely you are to succeed. Contingency plans also help insure success.
- Assess and categorize the skills you have learned in this program as follows:
  - —Physical ways of coping
  - —Emotion-focused coping
  - —Problem-focused coping
- In problem solving it is essential to have a variety of skills and to know when to use them.

Exploration Tasks

1. Of the three goals you wrote down at the beginning of this chapter, you have analyzed one in the exercises included in the chapter text. Now analyze the other two goals.

   Goal: _____

   Emotion: _____

   Self-talk (a.k.a. emotional hook): _____

   _____

   Cognitive distortion: _____

   _____

   Challenges to self-talk: _____

   _____

   Other skills you might use to cope with the emotional hook (for example, assertiveness, RR techniques): (Note that this was *not* part of the original analysis in the chapter text, but respond in terms of what you have learned about the different types of coping skills.)

   _____

   _____

   _____

Steps to take to solve problem or reach goal (be as specific as you can):

A. _____

   • _____

   • _____

   • _____

B. _____

   • _____

   • _____

   • _____

C. _____

   • _____

   • _____

   • _____

D. _____

   • _____

   • _____

   • _____

* * *

Goal: _____

Emotion: _____

Self-talk (a.k.a. emotional hook): _____

_____

Cognitive distortion: _____

_____

Challenges to self-talk: _____

_____

Other skills you might use to cope with the emotional hook (for example, assertiveness, RR techniques): _____

_____

_____

Steps to take to solve problem or reach goal (be as specific as you can):

A. _____

   • _____

   • _____

   • _____

B. _____
- _____
- _____
- _____

C. _____
- _____
- _____
- _____

D. _____
- _____
- _____
- _____

2. Draw a picture of yourself with crayons or colored pencils on the following page. Do not look at your earlier drawing (see Chapter 1) until after you have completed your second drawing. Do you notice any differences? What are they?

Supplementary Reading

Americans with Disabilities Act Handbook (Washington, DC: Equal Employment Opportunity Commission, 1992) [Employment resources; additional information at *www.disabilityinfo.gov*.]

Christopher W. Hoenig, *The Problem Solving Journey: Your Guide to Making Decisions and Getting Results* (New York: Basic Books, 2000).

Adam Kahane and Peter M. Senge, *Solving Tough Problems: An Open Way of Talking, Listening, and Creating New Realities* (San Francisco: Berrett-Koehler, 2007).

Richard S. Lazarus and Susan Folkman, *Stress, Appraisal, and Coping* (New York: Springer, 1984).

Use the space on the facing page to draw a picture of yourself.

10

The End of the Beginning

This is not the end. It is not even the beginning of the end.
But it is the end of the beginning.

—*Winston Churchill*

This book presents a great deal of material. There is no one place you should be at this point. Much of the work that you have done will stay with you and grow as your life evolves. Many graduates of this program have told me that it took about 6 months before they were confident about the changes they had begun. Continued skills practice, periodically reviewing the book, and staying connected with supportive friends and family all helped sustain the gains they had made. Many continued learning by reading the materials listed in the "Supplementary Reading" sections (see also Bibliography).

I also practice the various skills in this book. Although life continues to present me with challenges, I have more control in how I respond and that has made all the difference. For almost all who have worked with this program, pain remains a presence. Most of them, however, have established (or at least begun to establish) satisfying and fulfilled lives beyond the pain.

Relapse Prevention

During your good periods, it is important to think ahead about how to handle the more difficult times. This kind of planning is called "relapse prevention." It helps to keep a relapse from happening or keeps it short-lived if it does.

After people have started to use coping skills in managing their pain, they sometimes have a "honeymoon period" in which things aren't so bad. At those times, pacing or the RR techniques may not be practiced as regularly. Or the pain may get pretty bad, and people get discouraged again that "nothing will work." So they give up because they feel "it should be better by now." There may be other barriers to continuing with these new skills: lack of encouragement from those around them, increased personal stress, increased pain, additional health problems, "time constraints," or "inconvenience." All of these problems have been addressed in this book, but change in behavior is a process of forward steps and periodic retreats. Our research found that people with chronic pain who completed the program and believed they could manage their pain had less depression and less pain, and were less disabled. Working with the materials in this book can help you become effective in managing your own pain. That includes anticipating the problems that might confront you and planning ahead now to cope with them.

Make a list of what might get in the way of your continuing with the skills you have learned in this book. List those on the "Problem" lines below. Then for each problem, consider how you could get yourself back on track. The skills you learned in setting achievable goals will help here.

Example:

Problem: No one with whom to share the successes and difficulties of living with chronic pain.

Solution: Join a support group, keep a diary of your experiences.

Problem: Loss of a job.

Solution: Reread Chapter 9 on effective problem solving, contact vocational rehabilitation resource.

Problem: _____

Solution: _____

Problem: _____

Solution: _____

Problem: _____

Solution: _____

Coping with Pain during a Flare-Up

When the pain flares up or a crisis occurs, you may forget some of what you have learned. It's easy to slip into old habits when we are feeling out of control, even if these habits have not served us well in the past. For many people, pain flare-ups are inevitable and difficult.

In spite of this program's emphasis on the chronic nature of pain, many people expect that things should be better and that pain will not get worse after their hard work. They are unhappy to find that this is not the case. The nature of chronic pain is complex; the normal course is for the pain to have periodic increases and decreases. You may or may not be able to predict these. Where you have control is in your response to the pain increase. You can limit your distress by applying the comfort measures in this book to keep the pain at more tolerable levels. You can adjust your activities to reduce the discomfort you feel. Unless a disease or underlying process (nerve damage) has progressed, the great majority of chronic pain flare-ups are short-lived. They are just variations in the "volume control" of the pain system.

There are two ways to plan ahead for coping with pain flare-ups. The first is to plan for stages of increased pain. The second is to create a panic plan.

Coping with the Stages of Pain

To prepare for pain flare-ups, write down your coping plan for three pain levels: routine daily management, mild to moderate pain increases, and severe pain increases. Make a copy of this plan and give it to your health care professional. For example:

Daily Management

1. Medication: Pregabalin 50 mg three times a day, amitriptyline 100 mg at bedtime
2. Daily stretching, pool aerobics three times per week
3. Daily RR practice

Mild to Moderate Pain Increase

1. Heat or ice for comfort
2. Transcutaneous nerve stimulator (TENS)
3. Muscle relaxant
4. Call a friend

Severe Pain Increase

1. Reduce activities
2. Watch a favorite movie
3. Increase pregabalin to 100 mg three times a day over a week
4. Ice massage

Now it's your turn:

Daily Management

_____

_____

_____

Mild to Moderate Pain Increase

_____

_____

_____

Severe Pain Increase

_____

_____

_____

Panic Plan

The second way to plan for pain flare-ups is to develop a "panic plan." In other words, instead of panicking when pain increases, you can refer to a detailed master list of things for helping the mind, body, and spirit. To make the plan, list the options, skills, and techniques you have. *Be as specific as you can.* The more specific, the easier it will be to follow. For example, if you say "Call a friend," then add a detail such as "Mary Smith's phone number is 888-0983." Or if you say "Relax," add more specific details on how to relax (for example, "Do breath focusing," "Take a bath with lavender bath salts," or "Watch my favorite sport on TV").

Later, during a flare-up, you'll be able to refer to this list and know exactly what to do without thinking. Creating the list is also a good way of reviewing the coping skills you have learned. Don't limit your list to your new skills and techniques; also include older steps that worked to ease your discomfort, such as applying ice or heat and using medication.

For my mind . . .

1. RR technique—guided imagery

2. _____

3. _____

4. _____

For my body . . .

1. Hot shower

2. _____

3. _____

4. _____

For my spirit . . .

1. Call my friend John 222-444-5555

2. _____

3. _____

4. _____

Make copies of this list to carry with you, put on your refrigerator door, and/or keep in the glove compartment of your car. In other words, keep the list handy in various places for quick reference.

Now that you've completed your list, refer to the end of Chapter 1, where you were asked to write a similar list of things you did when the pain got worse. Do you find that things have changed?

A Celebration!

This program should end with a celebration. If you are in a group, poems can be read or exchanged, thank-yous expressed to other members, music played, and/or festive food shared.

If you are not in a group, take a moment and close your eyes. Imagine yourself in a room full of people. You realize that these people are strangers, but there is a sense of a common purpose and struggle. The room is vibrant with laughter, smells of food, and animated conversations—conversations about successful pacing of activities, who was assertive with whom, and recent pleasurable activities. Slowly, you realize that these people have just read the same book and worked with the same pain program you have been exploring. By your efforts and hard work, you have become part of a large group of people who have chosen to take an active role in their pain management. Enjoy your celebration with your imaginary colleagues, or, alternatively, give yourself the opportunity to enjoy the glow of a job well done. Reward yourself by going out to dinner with a friend, treating yourself to a getaway weekend or vacation, buying yourself some flowers, or all of the above!

Here are four examples of poems or other materials shared by program participants; all speak to the struggles, the courage, and the triumphs of individuals in chronic pain. At the end of the chapter, space is provided for *you* to write and express your thoughts to your unseen colleagues. A special thanks to all of you for sharing your experience.

Journey

I do not wish to be
as the log in a hot fire,
burning and raging
against its inevitable
fall to ashes.

I wish to be
as the pebble at an ocean;
washed and molded
by the waves and the sand,
warmed by the sun,
lifted by the tide,
everchanging.

—*S. E. Long*

Given

I will open this gift of pain,
Loosen its cords of rage,
Unfold the wrap of sorrow.

Is it a garment? I shall put it on
And disappear at once from sight.
(How much invisibility can I endure?)

I think it is an iron yoke of discipline,
It rings with authority:
My will must learn its place.

There is more, there is
Admission to another University.
Hard lessons.
Every leaf in the world
Must thirst before it falls.
Each predator becomes another's prey.
The mountain melts, earth labors.
Stars too must burn.
This little pandemonium in my brain
Opens a wide door.
To bear pain is to dance in holy fire
With Shiva the Unmaker
Who turns and turns forever his bright clay.
The gift of pain is knowing,
Knowing: it is so.

—*Margo Harvey*

A Gift from the Wish List

The door to the elevator was being held open for me as I stepped in.

"Thanks," I said before I realized it was he who provided the courtesy. Alone with just our reflections against the polished door, I felt I had to break the awkward silence.

"Excuse me, but don't I . . ."

"Bruce? Well I'll be darned! How are you?"

"Oh, just fine," I lied. "And you?"

I already knew the answer. I had seen him for the last two weeks in my chronic pain management course, but something had kept me from walking right up and saying hello. Maybe I wasn't really sure it was him, it had been so long.

"God, let me look at you!" he said, yanking off my ever-present cap.

"Hair's looking pretty thin," he chided.

"And you've put on a few pounds, I see," I countered. "No wonder I didn't recognize you in class."

The door opened at the ground floor, mercifully ending our mutual embarrassment at acting like strangers for the past two weeks.

"How long has it been?" I asked. "Can it have been fifteen years?"

"Almost twenty," he corrected, staring off as if surprised by his answer himself.

We spent two or three minutes standing there in the lobby, reminiscing about the old days. We were inseparable back then. Raised hell together and shared our secrets with each other. Then came marriage, careers, family. We lost touch. We had fallen off our respective Christmas card "A" lists, replaced by coworkers, bosses, and in-laws.

But everyone has a "B" list, a wish list, comprised of the names of people who really matter in life—names you wish you could keep in your life if only you had. . . .

"The time!" I gasped, looking at my watch. "Look, I've really got to go. I promised my boy I'd . . ."

"No problem," he said. "I understand. I'll be seeing you at class next week anyway."

"Until next week, then. See ya."

On the way home I realized how exhilarated I was at seeing my old friend, and that I didn't want him to remain on my life's "B" list.

I was able, with the help of my course instructor, to learn where he could be found. I looked him up the next day.

"It's good to see you," he said with surprise as he invited me into his living room. "Please, make yourself comfortable."

I felt kind of uneasy, as I'm sure he did, at this business of reacquainting ourselves. After a brief visit, I asked if I could drop by again soon.

"Anytime," he said, with a sincerity reserved for a true friend.

I took him up on his standing invitation almost daily, and before long I realized how these visits somehow helped my pain. Just like my weekly visits to the pain management class did. Only soon the visits with my classmates would end. I will miss them terribly, but I will continue to see my friend. All I have to do is post the sign:

PLEASE DO NOT DISTURB
I'M RELAXING PER MY DOCTOR'S ORDERS

—Bruce R. Comes

Thief

Alone, reluctant I entered the room
To sit among you
And become a thief.
Surreptitiously I observed your tears, listened to your laughter,
and heard your exclamations of recognition.

Furtively I gathered these riches,
Even as I slyly exchanged a shard of childhood joys,
A fragment of adult knowledge,
And placed your precious metals within a velvet purse
To carry in my exit unrepentant.

Perhaps you will forgive my theft,
Realizing at unresolved, unspecified future times
That I like an ailing, confused alchemist will spread
before me the treasures you presented and
Convert your platinum and gold to resurrected life and
rediscover with each revival what I stole:
The Release, Insights, Understanding, Security, the Comfort
To which
Your tears, your laughter, your exclamations
Have been transformed and stored.

Silently, I leave the room
My velvet purse no longer empty, I no longer reluctant, or alone.

—*Richard Cohen*

Thanks

Thanks for the wonderful trips to the beach—
It's given my mind some much-needed peace.

Even before this course, you see
I knew I was my worst ENEMY!

Anxiety, pain, depression too—
Similar to what all of you were going through.

I needed help; my patience worn thin,
The workbook showed me where to begin.

The weekly homework I did not shirk,
Mentally it was a lot of work.

How far I've come from that first day—
Looking at life in a whole new way.

Old beliefs discarded, changed attitudes I find
I'm doing my spring cleaning, but this year—of my mind!

So "thank you," my two teachers
And all the rest of you.

And as we leave I hear two voices:
"Remember now, you all have choices."
—Carol Rust

Now it's your turn to write a poem or a short prose piece:

APPENDIX A

Common Chronic Pain Conditions

Chapter 2 defines chronic pain in very broad terms as pain that lasts for more than 3 months. No matter what its causes may be, chronic pain has extensive biopsychosocial consequences. Thus the pain program presented in this book addresses body, mind, and the social environment. I respect the power of the skills and attitudes presented in this book. I also believe that state-of-the art medical evaluation and treatment must be included in the management of chronic pain. However, there is considerable misinformation and misunderstanding about chronic pain syndromes among health care professionals. Therefore, I want to comment below on some of the most common and least understood pain syndromes. I have chosen the particular syndromes discussed here for one or more of four reasons:

1. They are frequently overlooked, and an earlier diagnosis might reduce harmful treatments and psychological distress.

2. Certain aspects of their cause or treatment are not well known by health care professionals.

3. There are medical treatments, usually aimed at the abnormality contributing to the pain syndrome, that might help reduce the pain.

4. There are treatment regimens supported by new studies with high-quality evidence, including randomized controlled trials (RCTs).

A Word about Evidence-Based Treatments

Over the past several decades there has been an increasing awareness that physicians were not carrying out effective, well-researched treatments for many diseases, and that much of the treatment had very little research evidence to support its use. Part of the problem lay in the enormous amounts of information that clinicians and consumers alike have to wade through to find out what the research says. Until fairly recently there has been no systematic, organized way to approach the material. Multiple initiatives have been undertaken to address this problem and the Cochrane Collaboration is one such initiative. It has provided a methodical way of organizing all the research around a treatment or intervention question, for example, "Does drug A treat disease B?" All the available research is reviewed for that question. Then, based on an orderly analysis of results, the following conclusions can be drawn: there is good evidence to support using treatment A in disease B, there is no evidence that treatment A works, or more research needs to be done to prove effectiveness. Sometimes the conclusion is reached that the treatment is actually harmful.

These recommendations are based on the strength of evidence. Not all studies are equal. The strength of a study's findings is based on how well the research is designed and conducted. Research conducted as an RCT tends to yield strong, high-quality evidence. Other factors in the research that determine its quality include a large number of participants and a clearly defined set of measures to use in evaluating effectiveness of treatment. Studies designed this way most accurately test a treatment's success or failure. For example, a case study reporting that a treatment helped one person cannot predict if the next person will get the same results. However, case studies can be considered if a number of similar cases have the same result or if the result was dramatic in all the individuals. Case studies and other nonrandomized studies are used in developing treatment guidelines when RCTs are not available.

Fibromyalgia

Fibromyalgia is a chronic pain syndrome that affects primarily women (the ratio of women to men with fibromyalgia is 10 to 1). Encouraging progress has been made over the past decade in our understanding of this pain syndrome. We now know that it is one of many central pain syndromes and that after developing it individuals have an abnormally heightened processing of pain in the central nervous system.

Many terms are used to describe this syndrome, and overlaps among several of the terms suggest points along a symptom continuum. These terms include "fibrositis," "myofascial pain," "postviral fatigue syndrome," "chronic fatigue syndrome," "tension myalgia," and "generalized tendomyopathy." In 1990, the American College of Rheumatology (see Wolfe et al. in the Bibliography) developed the following criteria for the classification of fibromyalgia:

1. History of widespread pain.

2. Pain in 11 of 18 tender point sites on digital palpation.

For classification purposes in research studies, patients are said to have fibromyalgia if both criteria are satisfied. Widespread pain must have been present for at least 3 months. Many clinicians and patients feel that this strict definition of fibromyalgia, while important for enrolling patients in research studies, does not reflect the variety of presentations that can occur.

Many patients with fibromyalgia will also have associated complaints, such as sleep disturbance, headache, irritable bowel, irritable bladder, temporomandibular joint (TMJ) pain, chronic fatigue, painful menstrual periods, intermittent blurred vision, and short-term memory problems. Depending on the intensity of the symptoms, individuals with fibromyalgia may consult a gastroenterologist for irritable bowel symptoms and a dentist with TMJ pain, making the diagnosis all the more confusing. The presence of a second clinical disorder does not exclude the diagnosis of fibromyalgia, but the diagnosis is made many times after other diseases have been excluded (thyroid disease, lupus, rheumatoid arthritis, etc.).

The symptoms are quite variable and are marked by their intermittent, waxing–waning, and migratory pattern. This contributes to the long lag time between development of symptoms and diagnosis. The cause is unknown and is most likely the result of multiple factors. There is increasing evidence that supports a genetic predisposition, given that first-degree relatives have as much as an eightfold greater risk of developing fibromyalgia, compared with the general population. There are a number of environmental factors that are associated with the onset of symptoms, such as Lyme disease, Epstein-Barr virus infection, physical trauma, and emotional stress. These conditions may combine to trigger abnormal pain and sensory processing responses in the central nervous system. The two most consistent complaints besides pain are sleep disturbance and depression. It has been observed that the presence of depression does not appear to influence the sensory processing problems reported by individuals with fibromyalgia; however catastrophizing, a thinking style associated with very negative and pessimistic views of pain, does. Therapies directed at these two complaints can be helpful but not curative.

Treatment to date has focused on symptoms such as the sleep disturbance, pain, and fatigue. There is good evidence demonstrating the benefit of the old tricyclic antidepressants (particularly amitriptyline) in treating these fibromyalgia symptoms, presumably because of their ability to increase norepinephrine and serotonin in the brain. These chemicals are thought to be involved in pain modulation. Newer antidepressants more targeted to brain function, such as duloxetine (Cymbalta®), have been studied in fibromyalgia and are encouraging, but only for off-label use since they are not yet approved by the FDA for fibromyalgia. Antiseizure medications mentioned in Chapter 2 have also been used in fibromyalgia. Pregabalin (Lyrica®), an antiseizure medication that binds to brain receptors, has FDA approval for use in fibromyalgia. In an RCT reported in the *Archives of Internal Medicine* (Rooks et al. in "Supplementary Reading"), progressive walking with simple strength-training and stretching exercises was found to be beneficial for patients with fibromyalgia in a number of ways. Combining these physical programs with patient education and self-management provided both symptom and social/cognitive benefits. This study adds to the existing evidence in the *Cochrane Database of Systematic Reviews* supporting physical activities or a multidisciplinary approach to the treatment of fibromyalgia pain and function.

There are inconsistent results for research on acupuncture in fibromyalgia. In several instances increased pain was noted. This may reflect variability in causal factors such as genetics and sensory processing in the central nervous system.

In 2005, the American Pain Society released guidelines for managing fibromyalgia syndrome pain in adults and children. According to these guidelines, a synthesis of all the evidence available at that time, the use of medications, physical exercise, relaxation techniques, and cognitive-behavioral therapies is associated with improvements in pain, other fibromyalgia-related symptoms, functioning, and depression. Such a complex problem will not be improved without addressing mind, body, and spirit.

Many communities have support groups for fibromyalgia, and your state's Arthritis Foundation may sponsor such groups in your locale. The Arthritis Foundation also sponsors warm-water pool aerobics nationally. Information about these activities, as well as about fibromyalgia syndrome, can be obtained through your state chapter of the Arthritis Foundation. There are now multiple resources for information, support, and research opportunities related to fibromyalgia. The Fibromyalgia Network makes a good effort to report the latest developments and advocates for more research funding. Another resource for information and support since 1997 has been the National Fibromyalgia Association. Contact information for these organizations as well as other helpful links for fibromyalgia or for specific symptoms you are experiencing are found in the Internet Resources section at the back of the book.

Chronic Neck and Low Back Pain

Chronic pain in the neck or low back can be very challenging to treat. This is particularly so if no structural abnormalities are found, such as a herniated disc, a tumor (a common fear), or significant bony abnormalities of the spine (arthritis with or without clear nerve pinching or fractures). Repeated low back surgeries performed for complaints of continued pain often do not result in pain relief. This fact has caused many surgeons to recommend conservative or nonsurgical treatment if only pain is present. If no nervous system abnormalities are present in addition to the pain and if there is no evidence that a deteriorated disc is the source of pain, then repeating surgery may not be an option. More effective treatments should be developed as techniques improve for assessing dynamic (in motion) structural spine abnormalities and for distinguishing pain that originates from the different structures of the spine (facets, discs, nerve roots, ligaments, and muscles).

The Spine Patient Outcomes Research Trial (SPORT), a collaborative RCT, is beginning to answer questions about which interventions, such as surgical treatment, are effective, and for which back conditions. This is particularly important because of the potential negative long-term effects (including chronic pain) of having back surgery. These questions have not been studied in any systematic way in the past. Two studies were reported in 2006–2007. One concerned cases of degenerative spondylolisthesis (slipping of one lumbar vertebra on top of another) with spinal stenosis (narrowing of spinal canal), a condition that affects women six times more than men and is especially prevalent among African American women. The study found that surgery was twice as effective as nonsurgical approaches in reducing pain and restoring function for patients. The second study looked at cases of lumbar disc herniation with sciatica (pain down the leg). Both surgical and nonsurgical interventions were associated with improvements by 2 years. Although surgery may have had additional short-term benefits, the differences were not statistically significant. Look for more of these study results to appear in the future.

In the fall of 2007, the American Pain Society and the American College of Physicians published their clinical guidelines for the diagnosis and treatment of low back pain. There have not yet been enough good studies on chronic neck pain treatments to make clear recommendations for what is effective. The *Cochrane Database of Systematic Reviews* does report evidence supporting multidisciplinary biopsychosocial rehabilitation for neck and shoulder pain among working-age adults but states that more research needs to be done (Karjalainen et al. in "Supplementary Reading"). In any event, preventing disability from neck or back pain requires attention to both mind and body processes.

I have seen postsurgical patients whose pain was not coming from any surgically correctable problem, such as scar tissue pressing on a nerve or an unstable spine. It appeared to me that deconditioning of both the abdominal and back muscles contributed to the pain in these cases. In addition, poor body mechanics and misalignment may also contribute to abnormal mechanical force on sensitized nerves and soft tissue. A good conditioning program to strengthen the muscles of the abdomen and back can be very helpful. For alignment problems and poor body mechanics, I suggest short-term treatment with a manual physical therapist familiar with such techniques as myofascial release, Jones trigger point therapy, and muscle energy techniques. The Alexander and Feldenkrais therapies can be useful for poor body mechanics as well.

One of my frustrations as a pain specialist has been the realization that physical therapists and physical therapy treatments vary enormously. Physical therapy, like many medical disciplines, is very much an art. I recommend asking for a physical therapist who is familiar with treating chronic pain. This means identifying a physical therapist who is comfortable with the possibility of not providing total pain relief—one who can teach you about your body mechanics and how your body moves and who is aware of the importance of developing a long-term maintenance program that you will be able to do indefinitely. I do not expect the therapist to persist in treatment once you have stopped responding or progressing or if you do not do your home program.

Chiropractic treatment in chronic neck and back pain is controversial. It is unclear that it has benefits in long-term pain. But there is evidence that it helps acute back pain and flare-ups of chronic low back pain in some people. Chiropractic and manipulative medicine have been instrumental in stimulating the dialogue that is now taking place on the role of abnormal body mechanics in neck and back pain, particularly in those acute and chronic pain patients with no X-ray abnormalities (in the conventional sense).

Many chronic neck pain problems are complicated by what is referred to as soft tissue/myofascial pain. After traumatic events such as motor vehicle accidents and lifting injuries, many of my patients with chronic neck pain report not sleeping well, and they have multiple tender points in the muscles of the neck, on the tops of shoulders, in the trapezius muscle, and in between the shoulder blades. In addition to physical therapy that addresses posture and conditioning of the upper back and extremities, medication to induce restorative sleep can be helpful (for example, amitriptyline or desipramine). Limited trigger point injections with an anesthetic and/or steroids may be of benefit for initial treatment, and if there is evidence of facet arthritis (arthritis of the little joints that connect the spinal vertebrae), facet injections may also be of help. However, clinical effectiveness reviews of low back pain therapies reported by *Evidence Based Medicine* did not support proven efficacy for most injection therapies currently used.

Headaches

Headaches are a very common and disabling problem. Fortunately, most headache syndromes are intermittent. As in the case of back pain, multiple factors are possible as causes. Over the past decade there have been considerable advances in the understanding of headache causes. The old distinction between migraines (as vascular) and tension-type headaches (as muscular) is gone. It is believed that most primary headache disorders, such as migraines, cluster headaches, and daily tension-type headaches, come from disturbances in the central nervous system and represent different presentations along a continuum. If you are experiencing chronic daily headaches or difficult-to-control, intermittent migraine headaches, I would strongly recommend that you seek assistance from a headache specialist, usually a neurologist with an interest and expertise in headache management. There are medications that can abort headaches or reduce their severity. Evidence suggests that treating a migraine when it is mild produces a more complete and effective response than waiting until the headache becomes moderate to severe. There are a number of *-triptan* medications (for example, rizatriptan or sumatriptan) now available for alleviating symptoms of migraines. If frequent migraines are a problem there are also effective medication regimens to prevent them from occurring so regularly. Chronic daily headaches are also receiving more attention. A number of therapies have been found to reduce the incidence of daily headaches, and contributing behaviors have been identified as well. For example, avoid medication overuse, such as taking daily butalbital (for example, Fiorinal®) with aspirin, acetaminophen, caffeine, codeine, or over-the-counter medications for headaches. Medication overuse can cause rebound headaches; reducing overuse can reduce the chances of their developing.

There are several steps you can take to help you now or in preparation for your visit to a specialist. Keep a headache diary noting frequency and pain quality. Like the general pain diary, it will help you recognize patterns and triggers. Most effective headache treatments are categorized into prophylaxis (prevention), mild to moderate headache treatment, and severe headache treatment. If your headache pain diary shows regular use of caffeine or chronic daily use of acetaminophen, Fiorecet®, Fiorinal®, Esgic®, or other pain medications, then a large component of your headaches may be caused by rebound. If so, you need to slowly decrease the daily doses of such medication, particularly if using Fiorecet®, Fiorinal®, or Esgic®, since these medications contain barbiturate-like components that may be habit forming and may cause seizures if suddenly stopped when daily doses are significant. If you have any questions or concerns, consult with your prescribing physician. You should either limit your use of these medications to 1 day per week or not use them at all. Avoid long fasting periods during the day; this can help people prone to low blood sugar. Skipping meals is often associated with headaches in susceptible individuals. Finally, constipation may also be associated with chronic daily headaches. Increasing fluids, dietary fiber, exercise, and judicious use of stool softeners may help. More aggressive bowel regimens may be necessary for those using opioids (narcotics). Ask your health care professional for assistance.

When I see patients with complaints of daily headaches, I frequently find that they are suffering from muscle tension or spasm of their neck muscles. Variations on this theme are patients with TMJ strain caused by clenching or grinding of teeth, who typically have morning headaches; a night guard for the teeth may help in such cases. Therapy directed at strengthening of the upper extremities and good posturing of the head, neck, and upper back are extremely valuable, sometimes eliminating the problem altogether. If you experience increased headaches after exercising your upper extremities, you should take special care. You are probably using muscles incorrectly because of weakness and straining; get supervision at the beginning.

Interstitial Cystitis

Interstitial cystitis or painful bladder syndrome (IC/PBS) is a disease of the bladder that can be associated with stretch-induced hemorrhaging of the bladder wall. There are three key symptoms: increased frequency of urination (both day and night), pelvic pain, and increased urgency of urination. The condition is seen primarily in women, and the cause is unknown. The urine is negative for infection, although the symptoms of a chronic urinary tract infection are reported, and women may be treated for months to years before interstitial cystitis is diagnosed. The diagnosis is usually made by passing a scope into the bladder (cystoscopy), looking at the bladder wall for microhemorrhages, and taking a sample of tissue (biopsy). Treatment is available but does not always resolve or help the symptoms. A special study, called a systematic review, looked at the more than 180 different types of therapy reported from 1987 to 2006 (Dimitrakov et al. in "Supplementary Reading"). Because of poor study designs in most of the research trials examined, only the studies for pentosan polysulfate sodium (Elmiron®) were able to be analyzed sufficiently. They found that Elmiron® may be modestly beneficial for relief of IC/PBS symptoms. There are national and local organizations to support individuals with this condition and to keep them informed as to the latest research and treatment developments. If you have been diagnosed or have the symptoms listed above I strongly recommend identifying a urologist or specialist who is familiar and comfortable with treating interstitial cystitis. The Interstitial Cystitis Association (see Internet Resources section) provides names of health care professionals closest to you as well as more information.

Endometriosis

Endometriosis is present in 15–40% of women undergoing laparoscopy for pelvic pain. There is no correlation between the site or amount of disease and the presence of pain. Endometriosis is a disorder in women involving the appearance of uterine tissue (endometrium) outside the uterine cavity (womb). We do not know why the tissue becomes embedded in areas outside the uterus. The pain in endometriosis is thought to be the result of the microhemorrhages that occur with the monthly menstrual cycle and the resultant irritation of surrounding tissue. However, the number of abnormal tissue implants does not correlate with the amount, intensity, or frequency of the pelvic pain. There are most likely several mechanisms for pain production (for example, immune complexes that trigger inflammation and sensitization of pain pathways in an internal organ similar to that occurring in neuropathy). Treatments may vary from birth control pills to testosterone-like medications to hysterectomy with removal of ovaries. Such hormonal manipulations may be quite successful. There are cases, however, in which endometrial lesions may persist in spite of removal of the ovaries and in which pain persists after removal of both the uterus and ovaries. Repeated surgeries to cut and remove adhesions (internal scar tissue) rarely provide long-term relief except when they are extensive or associated with bowel obstruction. There are also national and local patient support groups and information resources for endometriosis. Resources and support are available through the Endometriosis Association or the Endometriosis Research Center (contact information for both in the Internet Resources section).

Neuropathies

Several well-known pain conditions are associated with nerve damage or nerve irritability and are thus known as "neuropathies." Probably some of the most promising therapies to date have come in the domain of neuropathic pain caused by damage to peripheral pain nerves. The following three conditions are notable for their intense, burning pain although other sensations like itching, numbness, or stabbing pain can also be experienced. It is critical to have a thorough evaluation by a neurologist or nerve pain specialist as there are many causes of nerve pain, including toxin exposure (alcohol, arsenic, lead), metabolic and inflammatory diseases (diabetes mellitus and rheumatoid arthritis), nutritional problems (vitamin deficiencies), infections (postherpetic neuralgia), and paraneoplastic syndromes (cancers associated with peripheral nerve pain).

Postherpetic Neuralgia

Postherpetic neuralgia and shingles are caused by the same virus that causes chicken pox, herpes zoster. The virus can infect any peripheral nerve during the recovery period from chicken pox and then lies dormant for decades, only to emerge as a painful skin rash. It is important to recognize its presence early because shingles can best be treated, and a chronic painful neuropathy perhaps prevented, if antivirals (acyclovir, famciclovir) are taken within the first 72 hours after the outbreak. The outbreak of herpes zoster is associated with a heightened sensation (hyperalgesia) of painful itching or skin discomfort from normally nonirritating stimuli (allodynia), followed by a small blistery rash that over the course of about two weeks becomes crusted and weepy. It may be associated with fever and flu-like symptoms. In individuals over 65 years of age, there is a high likelihood of developing nerve pain that lasts long after the rash has gone. Early intervention with tricyclic antidepressants and anti-seizure medications like gabapentin or pregabalin may prevent the wind-up of the central nervous system that is thought to contribute to the pain becoming chronic.

If chronic pain develops from untreated shingles then it can help to use anti-seizure medications such as pregabalin or gabapentin, amitriptyline if tolerated, or duloxetine to calm abnormal nerve firing. Another potentially effective treatment is to apply Zostrix® to the painful skin five times a day after the rash has healed. Follow the instructions in the box. Zostrix® is an over-the-counter cream made from capsaicin derived from hot chili peppers and is available without a prescription, but consult your health care provider to confirm the diagnosis. Some people experience intense burning upon applying the cream but after multiple doses this gradually decreases. A 5% Lidoderm® patch can also be applied to involved skin. The patch is applied for 12 hours at a time and then removed for 12 hours.

However, the best treatment is prevention. Recent availability of a vaccine (Zostavax®) developed to prevent the occurrence of shingles in older people and the ongoing vaccination (Varivax®) of children to prevent chicken pox will help make shingles and postherpetic neuralgia diseases of the past.

Painful Diabetic Neuropathy

In addition to causing a neuropathy characterized by numbness in the hands and lower extremities, diabetes mellitus is the most common cause of painful neuropathy. The risk for developing this condition is associated with increasing age, number of years diagnosed with diabetes, and poor glycemic (blood sugar) control, as determined by HbA1c (glycosylated hemoglobin) levels. There are a number of medications used for the treatment of diabetic neuropathy. There are first-line treatment agents, which have more than two randomized controlled trials (RCTs) to support their use in diabetes: duloxetine (Cymbalta®), pregabalin (Lyrica®), and tricyclic antidepressants (amitriptyline). Second-line treatment agents with evidence based on one or more RCTs in the treatment of diabetes or other neuropathies are gabapentin (Neurontin®) and carbamazepine. If pain is severe the opioid long-acting oxycodone and opioid-like tramadol are thought to be beneficial.

Complex Regional Pain Syndrome (CRPS), Type I

CRPS, Type I, is a condition marked by spontaneous pain that may be abnormally triggered (allodynia) or heightened (hyperalgesia), and is characterized by the "CRPS triad" of autonomic, motor, and sensory abnormalities. It has also been called "reflex sympathetic dystrophy," "Sudeck's dystrophy," or "hand/shoulder syndrome." The pain, which can develop after major or minor trauma to the extremities, is not limited to a single peripheral nerve and is often disproportionate to the inciting event; that is, severe pain might develop after a minor injury like an ankle sprain. The underlying cause of CRPS, Type I, is unknown, but the condition involves the sympathetic nervous system in the pain process. Symptoms include swelling, increased sweating, hair and nail growth changes in the involved extremity, and blood vessel constriction (causing the skin to turn dark red to blue, and cold) and dilation (which causes the skin to turn red and hot and to burn). Even light touch can cause excruciating pain. CRPS, Type I, is a very complicated syndrome and needs to be treated by pain specialists or, at a minimum, by someone familiar with the diagnosis. I mention it here so that if you have these symptoms but have not been diagnosed as yet, you can bring this description to the attention of your health care professional or to anyone you know who might have these symptoms. Multidisciplinary treatment must be done in a coordinated fashion for best results. Treatment may involve nerve blocks aimed at blocking the sympathetic nervous system. Best results are obtained if diagnosis and intervention are done early in the development of the pain syndrome. There is little evidence that surgical sympathetic neurolysis (permanent destruction of the nerve to the involved limb) is beneficial, but there is some evidence that spinal cord stimulation from an implanted stimulator may be beneficial. Medications used to help treat symptoms related to this condition are blood pressure pills (such as alpha-adrenergic blockers), anti-seizure medications (such as gabapentin or pregabalin—off label), and tricyclic antidepressants (such as amitriptyline or desipramine). Physical therapy, use of contrast baths, and desensitization of the painful limb are very important because they can help maintain function. A high-voltage galvanic skin stimulator may also help with pain and swelling. The scientific advisory board of the Reflex Sympathetic Dystrophy Syndrome Association (see Internet Resources section) includes the top professionals working on the disorder.

It should be noted that the treatment of all painful neuropathies can benefit from the management techniques described throughout this workbook. All chronic pain sufferers deserve treatment that addresses the needs of the whole person. But in neuropathies, medications and the other interventions named above are very important, since they can reduce pain stimulus intensity.

Supplementary Reading

American College of Physicians and the American Pain Society, "Diagnosis and Treatment of Low Back Pain: A Joint Clinical Practice Guideline from the American College of Physicians and the American Pain Society," *Annals of Internal Medicine, 147*: 478–491, 2007.

American Pain Society, *Guideline for the Management of Fibromyalgia Pain Syndrome in Adults and Children*, APS Clinical Practice Guidelines Series, No. 4 (Glenview, IL: American Pain Society, 2005).

Robert Badgett, "Review: Injection Treatment Is Not Better than Placebo for Relieving Pain in Benign Chronic Low Back Pain," *Evidence-Based Medicine Online, 5*: 121, 2000. (Accessed 4/27/08)

Jordan Dimitrakov, Kurt Kroenke, William D. Steers, Charles Berde, David Zurakowski, Michael R. Freeman, et al., "Pharmacologic Management of Painful Bladder Syndrome/Interstitial Cystitis," *Archives of Internal Medicine, 167*(18): 1922–1929, 2007.

R. A. Karjalainen, A. Malmivaara, M. van Tulder, R. Roine, M. Jauhiainen, H. Hurri, et al., "Multidisciplinary Biopsychosocial Rehabilitation for Neck and Shoulder Pain among Working Age Adults," *Cochrane Database of Systemic Reviews, 2*, CD002194, 2003.

A. M. Pearson, E. A. Blood, J. W. Frymoyer, H. Herkowitz, W. A. Abdu, R. Woodward, et al., "SPORT Lumbar Intervertebral Disk Herniation and Back Pain: Does Treatment, Location, or Morphology Matter?" *Spine, 33*(4): 428–435, 2008.

Daniel S. Rooks, Shiva Gautam, Matthew Romeling, Martha L. Cross, Diana Stratigakis, Brittany Evans, et al., "Group Exercise, Education, and Combination Self-Management in Women with Fibromyalgia: A Randomized Trial," *Archives of Internal Medicine, 167*(20): 2192–2200, 2007.

J. N. Weinstein, T. D. Tosteson, J. D. Lurie, A. N. Tosteson, E. Blood, B. Hanscom, et al., "Surgical versus Nonsurgical Therapy for Lumbar Spinal Stenosis," *New England Journal of Medicine, 358*(8): 794–810, 2008.

APPENDIX B

Complementary Alternative Medicine

The term "complementary alternative medicine" (CAM) has been used to mean anything outside of the traditionally Western high-tech, pharmaceutical medical system. According to the definition offered on the website of the National Center for Complementary and Alternative Medicine (*nccam.nih.gov/health/whatiscam*), "CAM is a group of diverse medical and health care systems, practices, and products that are not presently considered to be part of conventional medicine." A further distinction is made between complementary medicine, which is used along with traditional medical therapies, and alternative medicine, which is used in place of traditional medicine.

There has been considerable confusion about what works and how and when to use such therapies. It is only in the last decade that research methods and systematic reviews have been applied to them. The results continue to be of limited use because of poor study design, but there have been efforts to improve the quality, and hopefully the results, of this research. This entire workbook could be called an "alternative, complementary" approach to pain management because it is based on many of the therapies considered to be CAM therapies, such as mind–body therapy, relaxation techniques, and self-help therapies. The power of such therapies is the healing that they can promote: healing in the sense of finding comfort, joy, and purpose in living with a problem such as chronic pain.

There are additional CAM therapies that are similar to Western medical therapies, such as acupuncture and drug treatments in the form of biological agents and herbs. These additional therapies may reduce symptoms, though they do not cure the underlying disease.

Acupuncture

Traditional acupuncture involves the insertion of slender needles into specific points on the body. The needles may be heated with an herb (a process called moxibustion) or electrified. The rationale for point selection is based on numerous interpretations, and you may find an acupuncturist who describes his or her therapy in terms of nationality (for example, Chinese, Japanese, French, or Korean) or energy system (five elements, *Qi* [*chi*]). Many people find that acupuncture reduces tension and pain flare-ups and increases energy. There is some research indicating that acupuncture may safely reduce neck, low back, and fibromyalgia pain and pain in the knees from osteoarthritis. However, some patients with fibromyalgia may be very sensitive to needling techniques and will not be able to tolerate acupuncture. More studies with better methods are under way to further clarify what works.

Treatment by a licensed or certified acupuncturist may assist you with symptom control. Many acupuncturists use disposable needles to reduce risk of infection. In general, some improvement in symptoms would be expected after 8 to 12 treatment sessions.

The website of the National Center for Complementary and Alternative Medicine (see the Internet Resources section at the back of the book) is an excellent resource for accurate information on acupuncture and for the latest results of research trials.

Biological Agents

Biological agents are similar to those that are already synthesized in the body. The ones discussed here are glucosamine, chondroitin 4-sulfate, and SAMe. Although these agents have been promoted for treatment of pain, none has yet been approved by the Food and Drug Administration (FDA). This means that the optimum dosage for therapeutic effectiveness has not been fully researched. As a result, the preparations vary widely in the amount of active ingredient they contain, and long-term side effects (in years) are unknown (though Europeans have been using such remedies for years).

Glucosamine

Glucosamine sulfate is derived from chitin (the shells of shrimp, lobster, or crab) or synthesized. Evidence exists that glucosamine sulfate can decrease osteoarthritis pain and may stimulate cartilage production. The most frequently used oral dosage is 500 mg three times a day for at least 2 months. Side effects are rare and usually involve nausea or indigestion.

Chondroitin 4-Sulfate

Chondroitin 4-sulfate is a glycosaminoglycan, a component of cartilage. Supplements are derived from the cartilage of cattle or sharks. Evidence exists that chondroitin 4-sulfate taken at doses of 400 mg three times a day for 2 or 3 months can decrease pain in osteoarthritis. It may also slow cartilage breakdown. Side effects are rare and usually involve nausea or indigestion. Chondroitin 4-sulfate is structurally similar to blood thinners. Caution: If you are taking prescribed blood thinners check with your doctor before taking this. Many supplement preparations contain both glucosamine and chondroitin 4-sulfate.

In February 2006, the first results of the Glucosamine/Chondroitin Arthritis Intervention Trial (GAIT) Study were published in the *New England Journal of Medicine* (Clegg et al., in "Supplemental Reading"). In general, patients treated with chondroitin 4-sulfate and glucosamine did not achieve relief from osteoarthritis pain. An exception was seen in a small subgroup of patients with moderate to severe pain who did show significant relief with the combined supplements. This study will next assess whether there are reductions in disease progression, determined by X-rays of the knees, as a result of the glucosamine and chondroitin 4-sulfate treatment.

SAMe

SAMe, or *S*-adenosylmethionine, is a naturally occurring compound synthesized from the amino acid L-methionine and adenosine triphosphate (ATP). It plays a role in various metabolic processes and is possibly both anti-inflammatory and cartilage protective. It has also been thought to have a mild antidepressant effect. Several randomized controlled research trials (RCTs) have demonstrated pain reductions equivalent to those of anti-inflammatory drugs for up to 2 years with continued benefit in patients with osteoarthritis. Some people find SAMe helpful.

Herbal Remedies

Because of their widespread availability, millions of people have embraced self-medication with herbs in multiple preparations, from teas to capsules. Although most preparations are probably safe, some herbal compounds, such as those containing ephedra, an adrenaline-like substance, have been associated with illness and death. The active therapeutic ingredients in herbal preparations are like drugs. Many of our current medications had their origin in compounds isolated from plants (for example, digitalis from the foxglove plant, salicylic acid [or aspirin] from willow bark).

Some of the more popular herbs used by patients in chronic pain have been St. John's wort (for mild depression), valerian (for sleep), cayenne pepper (used externally, for anti-inflammatory effect), ginger (for inflammation and pain relief), and feverfew (for migraines). Kava kava has been used for sleep but has been associated with severe liver damage and is not recommended. St. John's wort has been shown to interact with multiple medications, decreasing plasma levels of certain drugs, for example, theophylline and digoxin. In addition, using St. John's wort with a selective serotonin reuptake inhibitor (SSRI) antidepressant (such as Prozac®, Paxil®) may increase the likelihood of experiencing "serotonin syndrome," marked by agitation, confusion, seizures, and tremor. It is recommended that you discuss the use of supplemental herbal remedies with your health care provider.

Several resources that can be used to explore the recommended use and effects of a variety of herbal substances are included in "Supplementary Reading." The Arthritis Foundation has very good advice about herbs and other CAM therapies in *The Arthritis Foundation's Guide to Alternative Therapies* (Horstman in "Supplementary Reading"). There is now a fourth edition of the *Physician's Desk Reference* available for herbal medicine. Current research into herbal preparations used in Chinese and Ayurvedic (from India) medicine may shed light on the active ingredients that make them helpful for treatment of a variety of symptoms. It is hoped that the FDA will implement standards for these herbal products in the next few years so that patients may know the safety and potency of available herbal preparations.

Massage

Many techniques fall into the category of massage therapy—for example, Swedish massage, acupressure, lymphatic massage, and reflexology. In these techniques manual pressure is applied to areas of the body to release tension in muscles, to prescribed points that are representative of body parts (foot/hand reflexology), or to acupuncture points (Shiatsu, Do'in, acupressure). Many people, with or without chronic pain, find that massage can help them release tension, treat flare-ups, or just relax. Some patients with fibromyalgia can only tolerate light touch, so it may be important to find a therapist with experience in treating patients with chronic pain and to use your communication skills for treatment feedback.

Meditation

In June 2007 the Agency for Healthcare Research and Quality (AHRQ) published its Evidence Report/Technology Assessment *Meditation Practices for Health: State of the Research*. Evidence was reviewed for five techniques: mantra meditation (Transcendental Meditation® [TM®], the relaxation response [RR], and clinically standardized meditation [CSM]); mindfulness meditation (Vipassana, Zen Buddhist meditation, mindfulness-based stress reduction [MBSR], and mindfulness-based cognitive therapy [MBCT]); yoga; tai chi; and qi gong. The majority of these studies were directed at the treatment of hypertension, substance abuse disorders, and cardiovascular disease. The study designs were of poor quality. As a result, this report concludes that "the therapeutic effects of meditation practices cannot be established based on the current literature. . . . Firm conclusions on the effects of meditation practices in healthcare cannot be drawn based on the available evidence." This is not to say that meditation practices do not have value. Rather, it points to the complexity of studying techniques that are subjective experiences when efforts are not made to standardize instructions, have clearly defined endpoints to measure, and have adequate controls.

Energy Therapies

Therapeutic touch, reiki, qi gong, and polarity therapy are all techniques based on alleged manipulation of energy fields. Although there has been no evidence that these therapies do more than help people deeply relax, many patients find the treatments comforting and helpful in relieving fatigue and tension. Many practitioners of these therapies also help their clients to reproduce the healing effects on their own, which can add to a person's pain coping resources.

Supplementary Reading

Agency for Healthcare Research and Quality, *Meditation Practices for Health: State of the Research*, Publication No. 07-E010 (Rockville, MD: Agency for Healthcare Research and Quality, 2007).

John Chen and Tina T. Chen, *Chinese Medical Herbology and Pharmacology* (City of Industry, CA: Art of Medicine Press, 2004).

Daniel O. Clegg, Domenic J. Reda, Crystal L. Harris, Marguerite A. Klein, James R. O'Dell, Michelle M. Hooper, et al., "Glucosamine, Chondroitin Sulfate, and the Two in Combination for Painful Knee Osteoarthritis," *New England Journal of Medicine*, 354: 795–808, 2006.

Ara DerMarderosian, Lawrence Liberti, John Beutler, and Constance Grauds (Eds.), *The Review of Natural Products, Fourth Edition* (New York: Lippincott Williams & Wilkins, 2005).

Joerg Gruenwald, Thomas Brendler, and Christof Jaenicke (Eds.), *PDR for Herbal Medicines, Fourth Edition* (Montvale, NJ: Thomson Healthcare Inc., 2007).

Judith Horstman, *The Arthritis Foundation's Guide to Alternative Therapies* (Atlanta, GA: Arthritis Foundation, 1999).

David Sobel and Robert Ornstein, *The Healthy Mind Healthy Body Handbook* (Los Altos, CA: Malor Books, 1997).

Andrew Weil, *Health and Healing: Understanding Conventional and Alternative Medicine* (Boston: Houghton Mifflin, 1998).

APPENDIX C

Working Comfortably

Nancy L. Josephson

Many patients who participate in the pain program work in offices and use computers on a daily basis. If you are one of these patients, correctly setting up your computer work area so that you are comfortable is very important in reducing or preventing the following:

- Neck and shoulder pain
- Eyestrain
- Stiffness
- Carpal tunnel syndrome
- Wrist pain
- Back pain
- Headaches
- Repetitive strain injury

Most larger companies are very "ergonomically aware" of correctly setting up work areas. If you are fortunate enough to work for such a company, take advantage of the services it offers. Even if your company does not offer ergonomic services, you can set up your own office so it is comfortable for you to work in.

Adjusting Your Chair

The best type of chair for office work is a "secretarial" chair (no arms) that has four types of adjustments:

- Seat height
- Seat angle
- Back height
- Back angle

Use the following guidelines when adjusting your chair:

1. Adjust the seat height so that your knees are bent at an angle of slightly over 90° and your feet are comfortable flat on the floor.

2. Don't cross your legs while working. That can constrict blood flow, causing tingling and making your legs "go to sleep."

3. Adjust the seat angle of your chair so that there is not a great deal of pressure on the part of your upper leg just above the knee.

4. Try to avoid chairs with arms. They put extra pressure on your arms and also position them at an unnatural angle if you tend to rest your arms on them.

5. You may need further lower back support than your chair provides. Ask your physician or physical therapist to recommend back support pillows that best suit your needs.

Adjusting the Monitor Height and Distance

Now that your chair is comfortable, move it to your desk and sit down. You're now going to adjust the height of your monitor so less stress is placed on your neck and shoulders.

1. Sit comfortably on your chair. Keep your feet flat on the floor.

2. Hold your head so that you are looking straight ahead, not down and not up. This is the position your head should maintain when looking at the monitor. Relax your shoulders and arms while you are doing this.

3. Raise or lower the height of your monitor so that you are looking straight ahead—neither up nor down. The monitor height should be approximately the same as your forehead height. You can raise the height of your monitor in a variety of ways:

   - Telephone books
   - Packages of paper
   - Catalogues
   - Specially designed shelving

4. The viewing distance from your eyes to the monitor should be 16–24 inches.

5. If the angle of your monitor can be adjusted, try tilting it 10–20°.

6. Once you have set the height of your monitor, sit down and see whether the position is comfortable for you. If you feel stress on your neck, try raising or lowering the monitor until it is comfortable for you.

Preventing Glare

Glare is the biggest single cause of eyestrain when a computer is being used. It is relatively easy to avoid eyestrain by following these suggestions:

1. Avoid setting your monitor in direct light (sunlight, overhead light, etc.).

2. Fluorescent overhead lights are the biggest culprits in causing glare. If possible, have the ones directly over your monitor turned off. You can always use a small portable light for desktop lighting if necessary.

3. Various types of glare screens are available at your local computer store. These can easily be attached directly to the front of your monitor.

4. Eyeglasses for glare prevention are also available, even for people who do not wear prescription glasses. Check with your ophthalmologist for suggestions.

5. Something as simple as a large piece of cardboard that extends over the top of your monitor can help reduce glare.

6. Avoid staring at the screen for too long a period of time. People who do this tend not to blink as often; this causes dry, hot eyes. Look away and focus on an object at a distance for a few seconds. Blink frequently to avoid dryness.

Adjusting the Keyboard Height

Carpal tunnel syndrome and repetitive strain injury have become fashionable ailments since the 1990s, thanks to keyboards and mouse devices. If you use a keyboard or mouse device, you are susceptible to these problems, but your chances of getting them can be greatly reduced by a proper keyboard height. Follow these guidelines when setting up your keyboard:

1. The table height of your work surface should be between 23 and 28 inches (floor to typing surface).

2. Use a comfortable wrist pad in front of your keyboard, so that your wrists lie comfortably on the pad instead of the hard tabletop.

3. Adjust the table height so that when you position your hands on the keyboard, your elbows are bent at a 90° angle and your wrists are not bent up or down. Make sure that your wrists lie flat and that your fingers are stretched out in front.

Using a Mouse Pad

If you use a mouse device, follow these suggestions to prevent wrist and shoulder stress:

1. Use a mouse pad to protect your mouse and make it easier for you to operate the mouse.

2. Try to move your entire arm when using a mouse. Many people make sharp, jerky movements with their wrists when using a mouse. This puts added stress on the wrist.

3. Take a "mouse break" every now and then.

4. Position the mouse pad next to the keyboard so you don't have to reach too far for the mouse.

Taking Breaks

If you spend more than an hour a day at your computer, the best thing you can do for your body and mind is to take breaks. Most computers have built-in clocks, and you can set an alarm that will tell you it's time to take a break. Determine how long you can work comfortably before you need to take a break. Then take that break!

Exercising

Exercising is also a good way to reduce stress while you are working at a computer. Here are a few exercises that you can try:

Breathing

Perform diaphragmatic breathing to help relax your body and to reduce stress and tension. Let your head relax along with your shoulders and arms.

Eye Exercises

1. Look away from your monitor and focus on an object at a distance for a few seconds.

2. Blink your eyes frequently to provide moisture.

3. Move your eyes to the left, then to the right. Look up and then down.

Stretching Exercises

The following exercises can help reduce any tension or muscle strain that occurs while using your computer.

Shoulders and Neck

1. Raise your shoulders toward your ears, and hold that slight tension for just a moment.

2. Relax your shoulders and arms.

3. Repeat this five times to prevent tightness in the shoulder and neck area.

Upper Back

1. Make sure you are sitting up straight.

2. Put your hands behind your head so that your elbows point out to the side.

3. Pull your shoulder blades toward each other until you feel a slight tightness in your upper back.

4. Hold this for about 10 seconds. Then release and relax.

Hands

There are two exercises for the hands. Here is the first:

1. Make a tight fist.

2. Hold for a few seconds.

3. Relax your hands.

And the second:

1. Straighten your fingers out in front of you.

2. Spread them as far apart from one another as you can.

3. Hold the spread until you feel slight tension.

4. Relax.

General Stretching

A good general exercise is just to get up from your desk and walk around, swinging your arms and moving your body.

Choosing Pain Medicine for Osteoarthritis: A Guide for Consumers

---

Fast Facts on Pain Relievers

- Acetaminophen (Tylenol®) works on mild pain and has fewer risks than other pain pills.

- Prescription (Rx) pain relievers may work better than over-the-counter (OTC) pain pills. They also have a higher chance of serious problems like stomach bleeding and heart attacks.

- NSAID pills, like ibuprofen (Motrin®, Advil®), naproxen (Aleve®), or aspirin, reduce pain but can cause stomach bleeding. You can lower your risk by taking the lowest dose you can for the shortest time you can.

- Aspirin can cause stomach bleeding even at low doses.

- Capsaicin skin cream, like Theragen® or Zostrix®, can help with mild pain. Capsaicin cream also has fewer risks than pain pills.

- Salicylate skin cream, like Aspercreme® or Bengay Arthritis®, does not work for osteoarthritis pain.

Choosing Pain Medicine for Osteoarthritis

What Does This Guide Cover?

This guide can help you work with your doctor or nurse to choose pain-relief medicine for osteoarthritis.

Reprinted from Agency for Healthcare Research and Quality Publication Number 06(07)-EHC009-2A, January 2007.

- It describes the different kinds of pain relievers.

- It also gives information about the trade-offs between pain relief, risks of problems, and the price of the medications.

This guide is based on a government–funded review of the research about pain-relief medicines for osteoarthritis. It includes over-the-counter (OTC) medications and some prescription (Rx) drugs.

Each of the medicines in this guide comes with benefits and risks.

- On the up side, they reduce pain and swelling. They can also help you stay active.

- On the down side, they may cause stomach bleeding or raise your chance for a heart attack.

People are different in how they weigh benefits and risks. Some people feel that a small increased chance of heart attack would be okay if they could get the pain relief they need. Other people would not want this kind of trade-off.

This guide can help you learn about the benefits and risks of pain-relief medicines for osteoarthritis. Knowing about the benefits and risks can help you decide what is right for you.

What Is Not Covered?

This guide does not include all the ways to reduce osteoarthritis pain. Exercise, losing weight, acupuncture, and surgery are some other ways to help you feel better and stay active. It also does not cover Rx opiate medications like morphine, Tylenol-3®, and Vicodin®.

Understanding the Benefits of Pain Medicines

Over-the-Counter (OTC) Pain Relievers

Acetaminophen (Tylenol®)

- Most people can take acetaminophen (Tylenol®) without problems as long as they follow the directions on the bottle.

- Research shows that acetaminophen (Tylenol®) reduces mild pain. It probably does not help with inflammation or swelling.

OTC NSAIDs

- Non-steroidal anti-inflammatory drugs are called NSAIDs (pronounced "EN-seds"). They include aspirin, ibuprofen (Advil®, Motrin®), and naproxen (Aleve®). These pills work by blocking pain enzymes.

- Research shows that NSAIDs reduce pain caused by swelling. They also give general pain relief.

- Aspirin is also an NSAID, but there is not much research about using aspirin for osteoarthritis pain.

Glucosamine and Chondroitin

- Glucosamine and chondroitin are supplements. They are not regulated as drugs in the United States, so their quality may vary. There is no way to be sure that the supplements you get in the store are as good as the ones used in the research studies.

- Research shows that the combination of glucosamine hydrochloride plus chondroitin sulfate may reduce moderate to severe pain without causing serious problems.

Skin Creams

- Capsaicin (pronounced "cap-SAY-sin") cream, like Zostrix® or Theragen®, is made from chili peppers. Research shows that it reduces mild pain. Five out of 10 people using it will have warm, stinging, or burning feelings. The burning feelings fade away over time.

- Salicylate (pronounced "sa-LI-si-late") cream includes Aspercreme® and Bengay Arthritis®. Research shows that salicylate cream does not work for osteoarthritis pain.

Prescription (Rx) Pain-Relief Pills

Rx pain pills include prescription-strength NSAIDs and opiates (morphine, Tylenol-3®, Vicodin®). This guide does not cover opiates. There are three kinds of Rx NSAID pills:

Traditional Rx NSAID Pills

- These are pills like ibuprofen (Motrin®), diclofenac (Voltaren®), and indomethacin (Indocin®).

- Rx NSAID pills are stronger and often cost more than OTC NSAIDs.

- Research shows that they relieve pain and swelling.

COX-2 Inhibitors

- Celecoxib (Celebrex®) is a kind of NSAID called a COX-2 inhibitor. It relieves pain as well as other NSAIDs do.

- Short-term research studies found that celecoxib (Celebrex®) is safer on the stomach than other NSAID pills.

- Two other COX-2 inhibitors (Vioxx® and Bextra®) were taken off the market in 2005 because they have a high risk of causing heart attacks.

Salicylates

- Salicylates, pronounced "sa-LI-si-lates," are Rx NSAID pills like salsalate, pronounced "SAL-sa-late" (Disalcid®).

- We do not know how salicylates compare to other osteoarthritis pain relievers because there is very little research.

Warning—If you have ever had stomach bleeding, high blood pressure, heart attack, liver or kidney problems, you have higher risk for serious problems. Talk to your doctor or nurse before taking any pain pills.

Understanding the Risk of Problems

What Is the Risk of Stomach Bleeding with NSAID Pills?

All NSAID pills, including aspirin, block enzymes that protect the stomach. This can cause stomach bleeding. It is not possible to predict any one person's risk. Research can't tell how long you can use NSAID pills without bleeding. In general, stomach bleeding is more likely for people taking NSAIDs who:

- Are older, especially more than 75 years old.
- Take higher doses.
- Use NSAIDs for a longer time.
- Also take medicine to help prevent blood clots, like aspirin or warfarin (Coumadin®).

Older people taking NSAID pills have higher risk of stomach bleeding

For people age 16–44:
    5 out of 10,000 people taking NSAIDs will have a serious bleed
    1 out of 10,000 people taking NSAIDs will die from a bleed

For people age 45–64:
    15 out of 10,000 people taking NSAIDs will have a serious bleed
    2 out of 10,000 people taking NSAIDs will die from a bleed

For people age 65–74:
    17 out of 10,000 people taking NSAIDs will have a serious bleed
    3 out of 10,000 people taking NSAIDs will die from a bleed

For people age 75 or older:
    91 out of 10,000 people taking NSAIDs will have a serious bleed
    15 out of 10,000 people taking NSAIDs will die from a bleed

---

What Are the Signs of Stomach Bleeding?

Call your doctor or nurse right away if you:

- Vomit blood.
- See blood in your bowel movement, or your bowel movement is black and sticky like tar.
- Feel very weak.

What If I Had Stomach Bleeding in the Past?

If you have ever had stomach bleeding, do not take any of the NSAID pills, including aspirin. If your doctor or nurse recommends NSAID pills, be sure to tell him or her that you had stomach bleeding in the past.

What about the Risk of Heart Attack?

NSAIDs can increase the chance of a heart attack. For every 10,000 people taking NSAIDs, 30 of them will have a heart attack that they would not have had if they were not taking NSAIDs.

Recent research found that:

- Some NSAIDs increase the chance of a heart attack:
  - Celecoxib (Celebrex®).
  - Ibuprofen (Motrin®) in high doses (800 mg three times a day).
  - Diclofenac (Voltaren®) in high doses (75 mg twice a day).
- Naproxen (Aleve®, Naprosyn®) does not increase the chance of a heart attack.
- We do not know how other NSAIDs compare when it comes to the chance of a heart attack.

What about Risk to the Liver?

Liver problems are rare with acetaminophen (Tylenol®) and the other pain pills described in this guide. However, taking too much acetaminophen (Tylenol®) can lead to liver problems. Be sure to follow the directions on the bottle. Keep in mind that other medicines contain acetaminophen (Tylenol®). Be sure to check the labels so that you do not take too much.

What about Risk to the Kidneys?

The risk is low, but all NSAID pills and acetaminophen (Tylenol®) can cause or worsen high blood pressure and kidney problems. Two out of 1,000 people stop their medicine because of kidney problems.

Sorting It Out

1. Benefit

The first step in choosing pain medicine is to sort out what kind of pain relief you need.

Do You Want to Be More Active?

Pain-relief medicine can help you keep moving. Start low. Use lower strength and lower dose pills for mild pain. Try capsaicin skin cream (Theragen®, Zostrix®) or acetaminophen (Tylenol®), because they have fewer risks than other pain relievers.

Do You Want to Reduce Swelling or Inflammation?

Try NSAID pills such as naproxen (Aleve®) or ibuprofen (Advil®, Motrin®). You can lower your risk of problems by using the lowest dose you can for the shortest time you can.

2. Risk

The second step is to know your risks for problems, like stomach bleeding and heart problems.

Have You Ever Had Stomach Bleeding or Were Told You Are at High Risk for Bleeding?

Do not use NSAID pills, including aspirin, unless they are recommended by your doctor or nurse. The best way to avoid stomach bleeding is to use acetaminophen (Tylenol®) as your pain pill, or use capsaicin skin cream (Zostrix®, Theragen®).

Have You Ever Had a Heart Attack or Were Told You Are at High Risk for One?

Most people can take acetaminophen (Tylenol®), aspirin, or naproxen (Aleve®, Naprosyn®). There is a chance of heart problems with other pain-relief pills, so talk to your doctor or nurse before trying them.

Do You Take Low-Dose Aspirin?

Aspirin, even at low doses, can cause stomach bleeding. If you want to take low-dose aspirin, consider a pain reliever that is not an NSAID pill, like capsaicin skin cream (Theragen®, Zostrix®), acetaminophen (Tylenol®), or glucosamine and chondroitin.

> Warning—Combining aspirin and other NSAID pills makes bleeding more likely.

3. Cost

The third step is to find out about the cost.

Is Cost an Issue for You?

Use the charts on pages 211 and 212 to compare the prices of different drugs. If Rx drugs are included in your health insurance plan, check with your plan about the cost to you.

Where Can I Get More Information?

For an electronic copy of this guide and materials about choosing treatments and medications for other medical conditions, visit this Web site: *www.effectivehealthcare.ahrq.gov.*

For a free print copy, call (800) 358-9295
Ask for AHRQ Publication Number 06(07)-EHC009-2A

For more information about osteoarthritis, visit the Medline Plus website: *www.nlm. nih.gov/medlineplus/osteoarthritis.html.*

OTC Pain Relievers*			Price for 100 pills or 1 tube***	
Drug name	Brand names	Strength**	Generic	Brand
Acetaminophen	Tylenol®	325 mg	$2	$7
		500 mg	$3	$8
Oral NSAIDs				
Aspirin	Bayer®, Ecotrin®	325 mg	$2	NA
		325 mg EC	$2	$5
Ibuprofen	Advil®, Motrin®	200 mg	$4	$10
Naproxen	Aleve®	220 mg	$7	$8
Topical creams				
Capsaicin	Theragen®, Zostrix®	60 gm tube (.025%)	$8	$12
		60 gm tube (.075%)	NA	$17
Supplements				
Glucosamine hydrochloride plus chondroitin sulfate		500 mg/400 mg three times a day	$55	NA

*This chart includes pain relievers from the research studies. OTC brand names are just a few examples of those sold in 2005.
**EC = enteric coated (helps prevent stomach damage).
***Average Wholesale Price from Drug Topics Redbook, 2006.
NA = Not available.

Prescription NSAID Pain Relievers*

Drug name	Brand names	Dose**	Price for 1-month supply***	
			Generic	Brand
Traditional NSAIDs				
Diclofenac	Cataflam®, Voltaren®	75 mg twice a day	$70	$160
		50 mg three times a day	$85	$175
		100 mg XR once a day	$85	$160
Etodolac	Lodine®	400 mg twice a day	$90	$110
		400 mg three times a day	$130	$170
Ibuprofen	Motrin®	400 mg three times a day	$20	$30
		800 mg three times a day	$35	$45
Indomethacin	Indocin®	50 mg three times a day	$65	NA
		75 mg SR twice a day	$130	$140
Ketoprofen	Oruvail®	75 mg three times a day	$95	$115
		200 mg ER once a day	$85	$100
Meloxicam	Mobic®	7.5 mg once a day	NA	$100
		15 mg once a day	NA	$155
Nabumetone	Relafen®	1,000 mg once a day	$85	$125
		1,500 mg once a day	$100	$150
Naproxen	Anaprox®, Naprelan®, Naprosyn®	250 mg three times a day	$70	$105
		500 mg twice a day	$80	$110
		500 mg three times a day	$120	$165
Piroxicam	Feldene®	20 mg once a day	$75	$115
COX-2 Inhibitors				
Celecoxib	Celebrex®	100 mg twice a day	NA	$125
		200 mg twice a day	NA	$200
		400 mg twice a day	NA	$300
Salicylates				
Salsalate	Disalcid®, Salflex®	750 mg twice a day	$20	$30

* This chart includes pain relievers from the research studies.
** XR/ER = extended release, SR = sustained release.
*** Average wholesale price from *Drug Topics Redbook*, 2006.

NA = Not available.

What Is the Source of This Guide?

The information in this guide comes from a detailed review of 351 research reports called *Comparative Effectiveness and Safety of Analgesics for Osteoarthritis* (2006). The Agency for Healthcare Research and Quality (AHRQ) created the Eisenberg Center at the Oregon Health and Science University to make research helpful for consumers. The Eisenberg Center developed this guide, and it was reviewed and tested by consumers.

APPENDIX E

Worksheets
and Other Materials

Contents

Sample Pain Diary

Name _____

	Describe situation ⟹	Physical sensation (0–10) ⟹	Describe physical sensation ⟹	Emotional response (0–10) ⟹	Describe emotional response ⟹	Action taken, including medications ⟹
Monday Date: 11/1						
Time 1: 8 AM	Breakfast	6	Achy	5	Frustrated	Shower
Time 2: Noon	Lunch	8	Throbbing	8	Disgusted	2 ibuprofen
Time 3: 9 PM	Bedtime	10	Sharp	10	Helpless	Heating pad
	Total:	24	Total:	23		
	Average:	8	Average:	8		
Tuesday Date: 11/2						
Time 1: 8:30 AM	Breakfast	9	Sharp spasms	10	Scared	Go back to bed
Time 2: 11:30 AM	Getting up	7	Throbbing	8	Sad	RR, heat
Time 3: 9 PM	Paying bills	5	Sore	4	Comforted	Paced activities
	Total:	21	Total:	22		
	Average:	7	Average:	7		
Wednesday Date: 11/3						
Time 1: 8 AM	Getting up	4	Sore	2	Relief	Gentle exercise
Time 2: Noon	Lunch	5	Sore	1	In control	RR, 2 aspirin
Time 3: 10 PM	Dinner out	6	Achy	1	Happy	Hot shower on return
	Total:	15	Total:	4		
	Average:	5	Average:	1		
Thursday Date: 11/4						
Time 1: 7:30 AM	Breakfast	5	Achy	1	In control	RR
Time 2: 1 PM	Housecleaning	6	Sore	2	In control	Sitting, paying bills
Time 3: 9:30 PM	Watching TV	5	Achy	1	Happy	Stretching
	Total:	16	Total:	4		
	Average:	5	Average:	1		

215

Pain Diary

Name _____

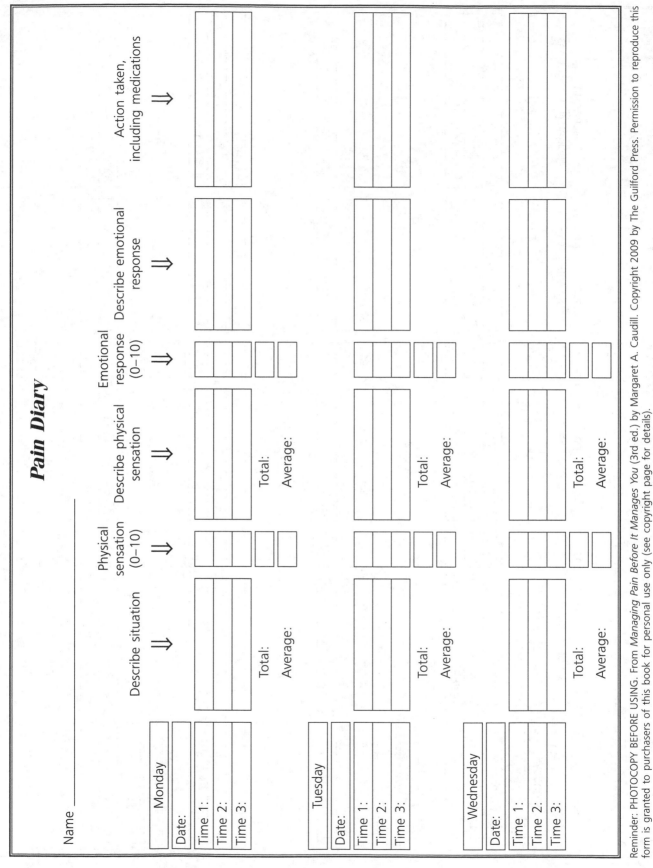

Columns (left to right): Describe situation → | Physical sensation (0–10) → | Describe physical sensation → | Emotional response (0–10) → | Describe emotional response → | Action taken, including medications →

Monday

Date:

Time 1:

Time 2:

Time 3:

Total:

Average:

Tuesday

Date:

Time 1:

Time 2:

Time 3:

Total:

Average:

Wednesday

Date:

Time 1:

Time 2:

Time 3:

Total:

Average:

Pain Diary (cont.)

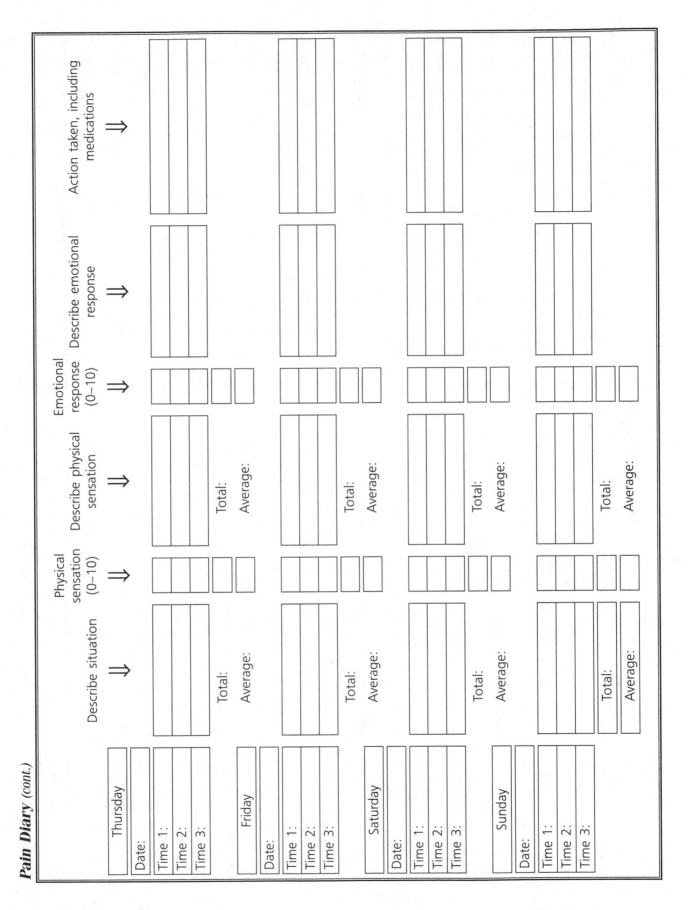

Medication List

Name _____   List last updated _____

Medication	How is it prescribed?	Pill dose?	Total dose per day	What's it for?	Morning	Midday	Evening	Bedtime	Prescribed by	Over the counter? (Check if yes)

See sample Medication List, p. 44.

Relaxation Response Technique Diary

Complete the following weekly RR Diary. Next to each category indicate the appropriate information about your daily practice. Use this diary for the first 3 weeks to reinforce practice.

Date							
Time started							
Time stopped							
Place							
Position (lying down, sitting)							
Degree of relaxation at end (0–10) 0 = very relaxed 10 = very tense							
Effects on pain? Decrease = D Increase = I No change = NC							
Method (tape, exercise, visualization, other)							

Were there any problems that prevented you from practicing the RR daily? How can you solve the problem(s)? _____

_____

_____

_____

_____

_____

_____

_____

_____

Increasing Activities Worksheet

Date: _____   Name: _____

Make a list of activities that increase your pain and those that decrease your pain (refer to Chapter 4).

| **Activities that increase my pain** | **Activities that decrease my pain** |
| Example: Washing dishes (standing) | Paying bills (sitting) |

_____   _____

_____   _____

_____   _____

_____   _____

_____   _____

Can you *delegate* any of the activities associated with pain increases? (For example, bringing dirty laundry to the washing machine.) Star (*) the ones you can.

Delegate one activity this week. It will be _____

Choose one "increase pain" activity from your list and time how long it takes to increase pain level by 2 points. Then choose a "decrease pain" activity and time how long it takes for the pain to decrease again. Alternate between activities that increase and decrease your pain.

Example: Pain ↑ Activity = Wash dishes   Pain ↓ Activity = Pay bills

Wash dishes (10 mins.)   Sort bills from mail (15 mins.)
Wash dishes (10 mins.)   Write checks (15 mins.)
Wash dishes (10 mins.)   Address envelopes (10 mins.)

| **Activity that increases pain** | **Activity that decreases pain** |

_____   _____

_____   _____

_____   _____

_____   _____

_____   _____

Can you *adapt* any of the above activities so that they can be performed more easily? What would be some of the adaptations? (For example: sitting to fold laundry or peel vegetables; lying down to call a friend or listen to a book on tape; opening cabinet door under kitchen sink so that you can rest one foot on the shelf; putting bowls in sink to stir ingredients)

_____

_____

_____

_____

Daily Record of Automatic Thoughts (Self-Talk)

Date	Situation	Automatic thoughts	Physical response	Emotional response	Cognitive distortion	Changed thought

Food Diary Instructions

Time started: The time of day that you begin eating a meal.

Food/beverage: Record everything you eat and drink. Note such things as whether the food or beverage contained a sweetener substitute or whether it was a new product for you. Are you eating five servings of fruits and vegetables and six servings of grain products (including whole grains) per day?

Quantity: The amount that you ate or drank (e.g., 1 cup, 8 oz. glass) or the plate portion (½, ¼ of the dinner plate).

Time ended: The time at which you ended the meal you were recording. (If a number of your meals last 10 minutes or less, maybe you should consider eating more slowly.)

You may have to keep a food diary for many weeks before you see a relationship between foods and pain patterns.

Food Diary

Name: _____

Date: _____

Time started	Food/beverage	Quantity	Time ended

Weekly Feedback Sheet

Name: _____

Date: _____ Reporting for week of: _____

1. Record the daily averages of your physical sensation and emotional response below:

	Day 1	Day 2	Day 3	Day 4	Day 5	Day 6	Day 7	Weekly average
Physical sensation:	____	____	____	____	____	____	____	____
Emotional response:	____	____	____	____	____	____	____	____

If this is your first session, record your pain level now (on a scale of 0–10): ____

2. Over the past week, has your *physical sensation*:

Improved ____   Stayed the same ____   Become worse ____

Why do you think that your *physical sensation* has improved, stayed the same, or become worse?

_____

_____

Over the past week, has your *emotional response*:

Improved ____   Stayed the same ____   Become worse ____

Why do you think that your *emotional response* has improved, stayed the same, or become worse?

_____

_____

3. List all medication you are taking:

Name of medication	Dosage (mg)	Frequency*
_____	_____	_____
_____	_____	_____
_____	_____	_____
_____	_____	_____
_____	_____	_____
_____	_____	_____
_____	_____	_____

*How many times per day or per week do you take each medication?

If you take opioids, how many pills did you take for this week? ____

4. Did you receive any other pain treatments this week—for example, nerve blocks, physical therapy, acupuncture, etc.? _____
_____
_____

5. How many times this week did you do the following?

   Relaxation response techniques _____   Mini-relaxations _____

6. For how long and how often did you do physical exercise this week?

   Aerobic _____   Time _____   How often? _____

   Stretching _____   Time _____   How often? _____

   Strengthening _____   Time _____   How often? _____

7. What goal did you set for the week? _____
   Did you accomplish it? (Y/N) _____   If you did not accomplish it, can you come up with a contingency plan that might help you succeed by identifying the obstacle and a solution to the obstacle?

Obstacle	Solution
_____	_____
_____	_____
_____	_____
_____	_____

8. Where did you find your pleasure this week? _____
_____
_____
_____

9. Do you have any questions or problems? _____
_____
_____
_____

10. To health care professionals: Is there any other information you wish to collect? Fill in before copying.
_____
_____
_____
_____
_____
_____
_____
_____
_____

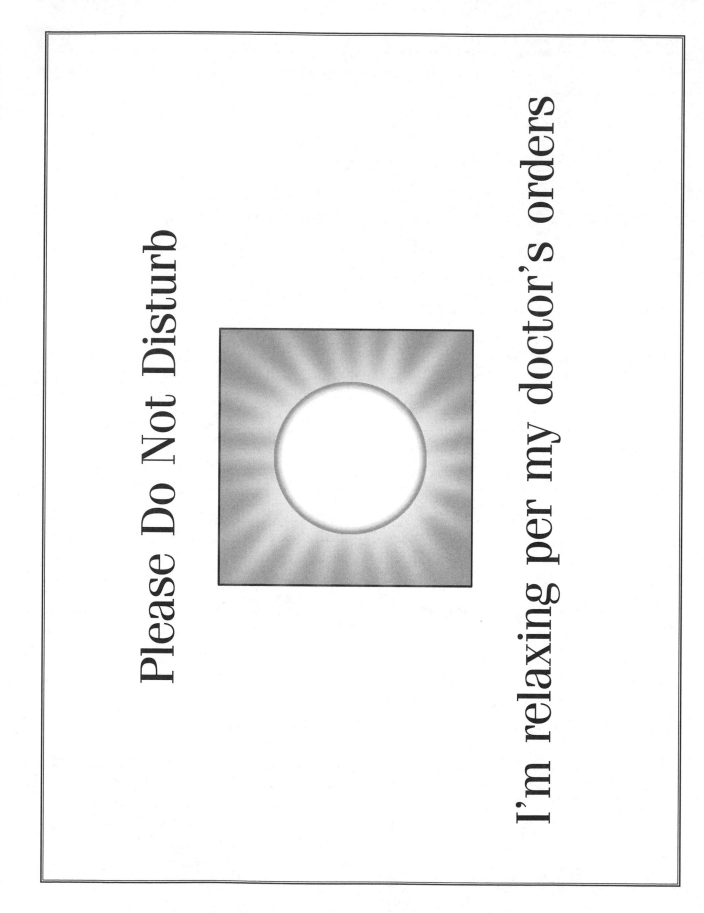

Please Do Not Disturb

I'm relaxing per my doctor's orders

Letter to Health Care Professionals

Dear Health Care Professional:

Managing Pain Before It Manages You is a practical, patient-oriented workbook. It provides information on basic pain mechanisms, medical treatment of chronic pain, and multiple cognitive behavioral skills that can assist coping and functioning. This book can be used by patients alone, but it can be even more effective if supported by a health care professional who can guide the patient through the program and reinforce the book's information. The workbook was originally written to supplement a 10-visit group medical program for chronic pain management, but it can be used in individual therapy as well.

If you are a physician, nurse practitioner, or physician assistant, this book can supplement the pharmacological, interventional, and surgical treatments recommended to patients with chronic pain.

If you are a psychologist, social worker, or nurse, this workbook offers a complete, self-guided cognitive behavioral therapy program for your clients or patients. It may be used in patient education, in conjunction with other medical therapies, and in psychotherapy. Patients can use the workbook independently or as a formal 8- to 10-week individual or group program.

Efficacy of This Approach

A growing body of evidence supports the biopsychosocial treatment of chronic pain. The biopsychosocial approach is further supported by evidence-based treatment guidelines such as those that can be found in the *Cochrane Database of Systematic Reviews* (*www3.interscience.wiley.com/cgi-in/mrwhome/106568753/HOME*), *BMJ Clinical Evidence* (*www.clinicalevidence.com/ceweb*), the U.S. government's Effective Health Care Program *effectivehealthcare.ahrq.gov*), and through such evidence-based search engines as the TRIP Database (*www.tripdatabase.com*).

The best approach to chronic pain syndromes is a comprehensive one that includes a thorough history and physical exam to understand the source of pathology or pain etiology, a stepwise approach to address the multiple sources of pain and distress, and repeated reassessment to assure responsiveness to treatment. Chronic pain is either perpetuated through central nervous system mechanisms (nonnociceptive) or related to underlying chronic painful diseases (nociceptive). Both types of pain are essentially incurable at this time unless the underlying pathology can be eliminated. As such, both are benefited by biological, psychological, and sociological therapies that reduce symptoms, increase activity, and assist patients in coping with chronic illness and managing their symptoms. The materials presented in this book are grounded in the principles of chronic disease management. They are a synthesis of medical and behavioral approaches to symptom and disease management that have been shown to decrease symptoms and decrease clinic utilization (Caudill et al., 1991; Becker et al., 2000). Furthermore, this intervention program can increase self-efficacy, an important mediator of pain-related disability and depression symptoms (Arnstein et al., 1999).

The Professional's Role in Facilitating this Program

> Those who do not feel pain, seldom think that it is felt.
> —*Samuel Johnson, MD, 1708–1784*

Progress has been made in the understanding of pain mechanisms but there is much that remains a mystery. While there is no objective measure of pain at this time, it is important to believe patients who report their pain experience. It is important for you and your patient to acknowledge that although living in pain is a challenge, there are many things that can be done to decrease symptoms and improve quality of life. If you do not feel comfortable evaluating and treating chronic pain, it is your obligation to refer the patient to someone who can.

Many health care professionals feel unsure about how to evaluate or treat pain. Such uncertainty has helped to drive the inappropriate prescribing of opioids in the past decade (Caudill-Slosberg et al., 2004). At the same time, there has been a dramatic increase in pharmaceutical advertising in popular media as well as to physicians. This has created unrealistic demands for pharmacologic cures by patients who understandably can feel quite desperate to be pain free. It is therefore crucial that the health professional and the patient understand the proposed pain mechanisms and treatment rationale described in Chapter 2 of this workbook. This information can help explain both the limits of pharmaceutical, surgical, and interventional therapies and the need for physical activity, good nutrition, and effective coping strategies.

Assessing and Encouraging Patient Readiness for Change

Teaching an appreciation of the biopsychosocial process at the time of the initial evaluation lends validity to treatments such as cognitive behavioral therapies. Explore what other symptoms patients are experiencing in addition to their pain. The professional can help identify stress-related symptoms such as fatigue, memory problems, irritable bowel, muscle tension, shortness of breath, palpitations, irritability, and insomnia. Questions about the patient's psychosocial history can help identify other influencing issues and provide more mind–body connections for discussion. For example:

- "What activities have you changed because of your pain?" Humans are incredibly adaptable and are quite capable of using denial for coping. Detailing what work and leisure activities have been curtailed inside and outside the home offers evidence for the magnitude of pain complaints.
- "Where do you get your emotional support? Who or what helps you to problem-solve?" Behavioral medicine research has documented the positive power of support through close friends, spouses, and religious affiliation. However, many patients with chronic pain suffer isolation and despair.
- "In addition to your pain and the problems it causes, what other stresses do you have to cope with right now?" This can be a very revealing question. The losses incurred from unemployment or decreased work capacity alone can have economic, social, and self-esteem consequences of enormous importance.
- "Have you ever been physically, emotionally, or sexually abused? Have you experienced a trauma?" There is a very high positive response to this question in my practice. Such histories are important to uncover since they influence how to teach relaxation skills. Patients with a history of trauma or abuse may require individual treatment to distinguish the emotional consequences of these events from similar experiences common in chronic pain patients, such as feeling vulnerable or out of control, or that one is not believed by others.

- "Do you have any fears or concerns about your pain? What do you think is going on?" The majority of patients have ideas (or fears) about the source or cause of their pain. For obvious reasons, addressing these concerns may go a long way in getting them to recognize their part in pain management.
- "What do you want to get from your visit today?" This sends the message that the patient has a right to have expectations for a visit. It is also a good starting point in clarifying unrealistic expectations. It can be the perfect opening to discuss the roles of the health care professional and patient in reaching a common goal.
- "If I can't cure you today, what would be the next best thing?" This question stems from a common response of many patients to the last question. They will say, "You don't understand, doctor, I don't want my pain, so why would I want to manage it?" This again allows for discussion of the nature and reality of chronic, persistent pain. Early in treatment many people feel that acceptance of pain management is a condemnation to a life of pain even if a cure comes along. They somehow think they will be excluded because they have accepted their pain. This misunderstanding is important to clarify. Acceptance is dealing with the here and now; pain may be mandatory, but the suffering is definitely optional.

These questions can quickly give you an overview of an individual's pain experience and lay the groundwork for establishing that pain is both stressful and affected by stress. It also sends the message that you are concerned about the pain and the person in pain. Listening to the patient's responses to these questions helps set up realistic treatment expectations and orients treatment to the patient's level of understanding.

Patients in precontemplation (Biller et al., 2000) who have not thought about the relationship between behavior and pain can be asked just to read Chapters 1 through 5 of the workbook, without doing the exercises described. They can also begin keeping a pain diary, as described in Chapter 1, which will help them focus on just how their pain is affected by their daily activities and mood.

Patients are most ready to start *using* this workbook when they can acknowledge (1) that changing their behavior may help them cope with or manage their pain or (2) that they need new skills to handle the physical, emotional, and cognitive effects of pain on their lives.

Guiding Patients through the Workbook

When patients are ready, this workbook can provide a guide for change. It is helpful to set a start date with the patient to begin implementing this program. It is also useful to review patient's goals. This demonstrates your interest and insures that the patient's goals are realistic and achievable.

Patients consistently report the benefits of the relaxation response technique, pacing activities, exercise, challenging negative self-talk, and diary keeping. If time is limited, focusing on these skills may be most productive. Otherwise, a chapter a week is a realistic pace to set.

With each week and each chapter, more observations and skills are added to the coping repertoire. Encourage patients to keep using and adding to the skills—with the hope of achieving a synergism—not just to do them one at a time.

To encourage action, ask at follow-up visits what patients are learning from their diary keeping, relaxation response techniques, and activity pacing. Because the cognitive therapy skills can begin to challenge some basic assumptions and beliefs, patients may be reluctant to do the writing exercises. These are crucial to changing cognitive distortions and ineffective patterns of thinking. Encourage patients to bring these exercise sheets to their follow-up appointments or to keep a journal. Journaling can help patients become more comfortable with what goes on inside the mind and how it reacts to the world. Growing self-awareness can gently move patients into action. This movement toward maintenance of action over time is essential for behavioral change to occur and set the stage for a new standard of living.

The sequence of chapters in this workbook reflects the way the program is taught. The arrangement of topics is geared toward encouraging patient adherence to the program through the gradual build-up of pain management skills. Techniques that are easier to learn and provide more immediate results—such as relaxation response techniques and exercise—are presented first. Once patients have successfully adopted these skills, they receive positive inducement to continue with the more complex techniques—ones requiring long-term practice, introspection, and self-reflection—taught in later chapters.

Pain Flare-Up Management and Maintenance

Chapter 10 of the workbook addresses relapse prevention and pain flare-up management. Whichever technique the patient chooses to employ, either "coping with stages of pain" or the "panic plan," a copy of the plan should be kept in his or her record and periodically updated. Referral to the plan can then be made should he or she experience a pain flare-up. However, if the patient insists that a particular pain flare-up is different from what he or she usually experiences, a reassessment is necessary to rule out other developments. I have found that once patients become active participants in pain management through this program, they are the best judges of their own pain experience.

From here on, periodic inquiries about maintenance of skills such as relaxation response techniques (Chapter 3), mini-relaxations (Chapter 3), pacing activities (Chapter 4), strategies for response to negative emotional states (Chapters 5 and 6), reduced caffeine consumption (Chapter 7), and communication skills (Chapter 8) will also serve to reinforce behavioral change maintenance. If patients have stopped practicing these skills and are having increased difficulty with pain management, it may be necessary for you to identify the specific problems holding them back. For example, has a setback occurred because the patient was secretly hoping this program would cure his or her pain, and it didn't? Did the patient stop the program because it was going so well it didn't seem necessary anymore? Or is a separate life crisis distracting him or her from the pain management program? Once you have determined what issues are involved, you can set a date for the patient to get back into the program and then reinstitute a schedule of periodic checks on his or her skills practice.

A Final Note

I cannot emphasize enough what a rewarding experience it is to see people change, improve their quality of life, and feel more empowered in the face of some of the most difficult pain problems. It is critical to start from where the patients are in terms of their level of information, beliefs, and readiness to consider new directions in behavior and lifestyle practices. Your important role in facilitating this process will have its own rewards.

Margaret A. Caudill, MD, PhD, MPH
Dartmouth Medical School
Hanover, NH

Letter to Health Care Professionals *(cont.)*

References

Paul Arnstein, Margaret Caudill, Carol Lynn Mandle, A. Norris, and Ralph Beasley, "Self-Efficacy as a Mediator of the Relationship Between Pain Intensity, Disability and Depression in Chronic Pain Patients," *Pain, 81*: 483–491, 1999.

Niels Becker, Per Sjogren, Per Bech, Alf Kornelius Olsen, and Jorgen Eriksen, "Treatment Outcome of Chronic Nonmalignant Pain Patients Managed in a Danish Multidisciplinary Pain Centre Compared to General Practice: A Randomised Controlled Trial," *Pain, 84*: 203–211, 2000.

Nicola Biller, Paul Arnstein, Margaret Caudill, Carol Wells-Federman, and Carolyn Guberman, "Predicting Completion of a Cognitive-Behavioral Pain Management Program by Initial Measures of a Chronic Pain Patient's Readiness for Change. *Clinical Journal of Pain, 16*(4): 352–359, 2000.

Margaret Caudill, Richard Schnable, Patricia Zuttenneister, Herbert Benson, and Richard Friedman, "Decreased Clinic Use by Chronic Pain Patients: Response to Behavioral Medicine Intervention," *Clinical Journal of Pain, 7*: 305–310, 1991.

Margaret Caudill-Slosberg, Lisa Schwartz, and Steven Woloshin, "Office Visits and Analgesic Prescriptions for Musculoskeletal Pain in US: 1980 vs. 2000," *Pain, 109*: 514–519, 2004.

Dennis Turk, Donald Meichenbaum, and Myles Genest, *Pain and Behavioral Medicine: A Cognitive-Behavioral Perspective* (New York: Guilford Press, 1985).

Internet Resources

A great deal of information, misinformation, and opinion is available on the Internet. It can be a challenge to sort fact from opinion, and what's accurate from what's not. Listed below are those Internet resources that have been useful to me and my patients and whose information appears to be reliable. However, things change rapidly, so you need to make your own assessment. Check out the information you find with your health care professionals and consult your local librarians, who can give you personal assistance. Let me begin with a few general tips on how to assess the accuracy and reliability of information you find on the Internet.

Is It Accurate?

Some websites are more likely to offer accurate information than others because of their professional, governmental, or institutional association. A few organizations have attempted to set up rules that promote ethical presentation of information—such as guidelines on including the source and purpose of information. One such organization is the Health on the Net Foundation Code of Conduct (HONcode) for medical and health websites. This organization regularly reviews those sites that carry the HONcode emblem to insure maintenance of its standards. It does not rate the quality of information.

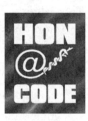

There are some simple checks that you can do to make your own assessment of information:

- Look for a recent "last updated" date. This is usually at the bottom of the home page. Information changes rapidly and a site that has not been updated in a year is suspect.
- Look for the site sponsor. This can usually be found as an abbreviation in the "address" or URL (Uniform Resource Locator) of the website. Take the following address as an example: *www.nlm.nih.gov/medlineplus*. The *nlm* stands for National Library of Medicine, *nih* is National Institutes of Health, *.gov* confirms that a major governmental institution is involved and should provide reliable information. If you access a personal website, exercise some caution in distinguishing fact from opinion. Personal websites often have a tilde (~) before the owner's name, but not always. You can find out who owns an Internet domain at *www.whois.net*.

- Compare information from multiple sources when available. Discrepancies indicate that there is a disagreement or inaccuracy, or that the material is opinion rather than fact.

- If it sounds far out or too good to be true, it probably is.

- Watch out for sites whose main interest is to get you to buy remedies and supplements or push their agenda—unless there is credible information to support their claims. If they don't provide evidence to support their claims and just say "trust us," then don't.

- Be aware that search engines use complex formulas for presenting the results of a search. Some search engines move those who pay more up front.

There are also a number of sites that give suggestions for evaluating online resources. Just do a search for "Internet accuracy" and you will see what I mean.

Websites for Health Information

National Library of Medicine (NLM)

Consumer Questions: *www.nlm.nih.gov/medlineplus*

This is a great resource for consumer health questions. Use the Index, look under *P*, and then look up *pain* for specific pain-related information. You can also look up information by the body area involved—for example, *back pain* under *B*—in the Index. Use this site to find all sorts of information about other health-related topics as well.

Medication Information: *www.nlm.nih.gov/medlineplus/druginformation.html*

This reliable resource is the National Library of Medicine's page for information on medication, including drugs, herbals, and supplements.

Medical Research: *www.PubMed.gov*

This site is a joint service of the National Library of Medicine and the National Institutes of Health. It can be used to search for published research literature on any medical topic, including pain.

National Institutes of Health (NIH)

health.nih.gov

This site is the consumer health information resource of the National Institutes of Health. Its home page lists a number of reliable health information links, many of which I have listed here.

National Institute of Neurological Disorders and Stroke (NINDS)

www.ninds.nih.gov/disorders/chronic_pain

This institute is part of the National Institutes of Health and is home to the "Pain: Hope Through Research" Web page, which provides excellent information about pain. On the left side of the page there is a link to *clinicaltrials.gov*, a site listing current clinical trials relevant to pain and other medical and mental health disorders, and their recruitment status.

National Center for Complementary and Alternative Medicine (NCCAM)

nccam.nih.gov

This agency is also part of the National Institutes of Health. Its website is a resource for information on herbal therapies, acupuncture, and other forms of alternative and complementary medicine. This site also has a list of clinical trials. On the home page, click on "Research," then on the right-hand side of the next page click on "Clinical Trials." Under "NCCAM Clinical Trials" click on "A–Z list of NCCAM Trials." Address: NCCAM Clearinghouse, P.O. Box 7923, Gaithersburg, MD 20898; e-mail: *info@nccam.nih.gov.*

Agency for Healthcare Research and Quality (AHRQ)

effectivehealthcare.ahrq.gov

Part of the U.S. Department of Health and Human Services, this agency has an evolving website with research information that is updated continually as treatment benefits and safety are determined by reports on multiple health topics. It is the site where *Choosing Pain Medicine for Osteoarthritis: A Guide for Consumers*, was obtained for reproduction in Appendix D.

WebMD

www.rxlist.com/script/main/hp.asp

This is home of WebMD's RxList, an online medical resource for detailed and current pharmaceutical information on brand and generic drugs.

HealingWell

www.healingwell.com

This site is a resource for patients, caregivers, and families coping with illness. The website features health articles, medical news, video webcasts, community message boards and chat rooms, clinical health care resources, e-mail, newsletters, books and reviews, and resource link directories on a wide range of diseases, disorders, and chronic illness. The health content is contributed by reputable health organizations, including the National Institutes of Health, Mediwire, e-HealthSource, and Healthology Inc.

Evidence-Based Treatment Resources

TRIP Database

www.tripdatabase.com

This is an evidence-based medical search engine. For example, you can put "pain" in the "search" box and be connected with published research articles that identify the best evidence available about treatments.

British Medical Journal

www.clinicalevidence.com/ceweb

While not free, the *British Medical Journal*'s clinical evidence website provides a resource for finding research summaries, guidelines, and best practices for any medical topic, with a pay-per-view option.

Relaxation Response Resources

Mindfulness Meditation Practice CDs and Tapes

www.mindfulnesstapes.com

This is the website of Jon Kabat-Zinn, internationally known meditation teacher, author, researcher, and clinician in the fields of mind–body medicine, integrative medicine, lifestyle change, and self-healing.

Amazon.com

www.amazon.com

Amazon has a wide variety of relaxation, meditation, and spiritual resources in book and audio formats.

Mayo Clinic

www.mayoclinic.com/health/relaxation-technique/SR00007

This page on the Mayo Clinic's website provides descriptions of various relaxation techniques. It also offers a few resources, such as a brief relaxation video with written instructions.

Cognitive Therapy Resources

Academy of Cognitive Therapy

www.academyofct.org/library/certifiedmembers

On this website, you can look for cognitive-behavioral therapists nationally and internationally, but not all states in the United States are listed.

Nutrition Resources

Tufts University Health & Nutrition Letter

tuftshealthletter.com

This is a useful newsletter with a reasonable subscription rate ($24/year in 2009—Internet offer).

Center for Science in the Public Interest

cspinet.org

The Center for Science in the Public Interest has been a strong advocate for nutrition and health, food safety, alcohol policy, and sound science since 1971. The organization publishes the *Nutrition Action Healthletter*, another useful newsletter.

U.S. Department of Agriculture, MyPyramid

www.mypyramid.gov

This website is home to the USDA's MyPyramid. Here you can personalize your own dietary needs and find more about the latest nutritional recommendations.

Harvard School of Public Health, Food Pyramids

www.hsph.harvard.edu/nutritionsource/what-should-you-eat/pyramid-full-story

This website presents a discussion of food pyramid history, the politics behind the pyramid, and Harvard's own alternative approach through the Healthy Eating Pyramid.

Oldways

www.oldwayspt.org

This website is home of Oldways, a nonprofit food issues advocacy group. Oldways programs are focused on nutrition (health, science), tradition (pleasure, joy, history) and sustainability (environment, organic). This site offers Asian, Latin, Mediterranean, and vegetarian pyramids that are good, evidence-based guides for healthy eating.

Glycemic Index

www.glycemicindex.com

The University of Sydney in Australia maintains a website where the principles of the glycemic index are explained and an updated searchable database provides information for over 1,000 foods from all over the world.

Pain-Related Web Resources

Nonprofit Pain Organizations

American Pain Foundation

www.painfoundation.org

The mission of the American Pain Foundation is to serve people with pain through information, advocacy, and support. Address: 201 North Charles Street, Suite 710, Baltimore, MD 21201-4111; e-mail: *info@painfoundation.org*.

American Chronic Pain Association

www.theacpa.org

The American Chronic Pain Association is a long-standing advocacy group started in 1980 by Penny Cowan for people in pain and their families. Address: P.O. Box 850, Rocklin, CA 95677-0850; e-mail: *ACPA@pacbell.net*.

Chronic Pain Support Group

ChronicPainSupport.org

The Chronic Pain Support Group (CPSG) provides a safe Internet environment where those living in pain can get the support they need.

American Pain Society

www.ampainsoc.org

The American Pain Society is a professional organization of pain specialists. It brings together a diverse, multidisciplinary group of scientists and clinicians. Its aim is to reduce pain-related suffering by increasing the knowledge of pain and its treatment and by influencing public policy. Address: 4700 West Lake Avenue, Glenview, IL 60025; e-mail: *info@ampainsoc.org*.

American Academy of Pain Management

www.aapainmanage.org

The Academy is an interdisciplinary organization of clinicians whose mission is to help people with pain through education, standards of care, and advocacy. Address: 13947 Mono Way #A, Sonora, CA 95370.

Headaches

National Headache Foundation

www.headaches.org

The National Headache Foundation works to improve health care for headache sufferers through provision of information, public education, and promotion of research.

National Migraine Association

www.migraines.org

This is the website of the National Migraine Association, or MAGNUM (Migraine Awareness Group: A National Understanding for Migraineurs).

American Headache Society

www.achenet.org

This is the website of the American Headache Society's Committee for Headache Education. ACHE is sponsored and directed by the American Headache Society, a professional society of health care providers dedicated to the study and treatment of headache and face pain. The site has patient education resources and referral options.

Endometriosis and Vulvodynia

Endometriosis Association

www.endometriosisassn.org

Endo-Online is the online resource of the Endometriosis Association. The first endometriosis advocacy group, it was started in 1980 as an independent self-help organization for women with endometriosis, doctors, and others interested in the disease. It has been a force behind innovative research on the causes and treatment of endometriosis. Address: International Headquarters, 8585 North 76th Place, Milwaukee, WI 53223.

Endometriosis Research Center

www.endocenter.org

The Endometriosis Research Center maintains a database of materials including educational sheets, videos, and newsletters. The organization advocates for initiatives ranging from research funding to maintenance of a patient registry and recruiting for clinical trials. Address: World Headquarters, 630 Ibis Drive, Delray Beach, FL 33444.

National Vulvodynia Association

www.nva.org

Vulvodynia, which is not specifically addressed in this workbook, is a chronic pain syndrome involving the female vulva that, like CRPS, Type I, and interstitial cystitis, is poorly understood but in need of patient support and validation. Address: P.O. Box 4491, Silver Springs, MD 20914-4491.

Fibromyalgia, Arthritis

National Fibromyalgia Association

www.fmaware.org

This is the website of the National Fibromyalgia Association, whose mission is "to develop and execute programs dedicated to improving the quality of life for people with fibromyalgia." Address: 2121 South Towne Centre Place, Suite 300, Anaheim, CA 92806.

Fibromyalgia Network

www.fmnetnews.com

The Fibromyalgia Network is an advocacy and support group for people with fibromyalgia. It publishes a quarterly newsletter. Address: P.O. Box 31750, Tucson, AZ 85751-1750.

Arthritis Foundation

www.arthritis.org

The Arthritis Foundation is an information and support resource for all types of arthritic conditions, including both common ones—rheumatoid arthritis, osteoarthritis, fibromyalgia—and not-so-common ones, such as Ehlers–Danlos syndrome (EDS), Marfan syndrome, and polymyalgia rheumatica.

Interstitial Cystitis

Interstitial Cystitis Association

www.ichelp.org

The website is brimming with resources, information, and treatment options. Address: 100 Park Avenue, Suite 108A, Rockville, MD 20850.

Complex Regional Pain Syndrome (CRPS) or Reflex Sympathetic Dystrophy (RSD)

Reflex Sympathetic Dystrophy Syndrome Association

www.rsds.org

Mission is to promote public and professional awareness of CRPS. Address: RSDSA, P.O. Box 502, Milford, CT 06460; e-mail: *info@rsds.org*.

American RSD Hope

www.rsdhope.org

This is a home-grown website with an assorted range of information for patients with RSD, their family members and friends, and other concerned individuals. Address: P.O. Box 875, Harrison, ME 04040.

Neuropathy

Neuropathy Association

www.neuropathy.org

This association was established in 1995 by people with neuropathy, their families and friends, and experts in the field. Its aim is to help those who suffer from disorders that affect the peripheral nerves. It is affiliated with seven neuropathy centers at major university hospitals across the country, which serve patients with neuropathy by providing treatment and conducting research into the causes and cure of neuropathy. The website includes a directory of support groups. Address: 60 East 42nd St., Suite 942, New York, NY 10165; e-mail: *info@neuropathy.org*.

Bibliography

This bibliography contains a complete list of all the books and articles recommended in the "Supplementary Reading" sections of various chapters, plus some additional resources.

Agency for Healthcare Research and Quality, *Choosing Pain Medicine for Osteoarthritis: A Guide for Consumers*, AHRQ Publication Number 06(07)-EHC009-2A. Available at *www.effectivehealthcare.ahrq.gov*.

Agency for Healthcare Research and Quality, *Meditation Practices for Health: State of the Research*, Publication No. 07-E010 (Rockville, MD: Agency for Healthcare Research and Quality, 2007).

American College of Physicians and the American Pain Society, "Diagnosis and Treatment of Low Back Pain: A Joint Clinical Practice Guideline from the American College of Physicians and the American Pain Society," *Annals of Internal Medicine, 147*: 478–491, 2007.

American Heart Association, *American Heart Association Low-Fat, Low Cholesterol Cookbook, 3rd Edition: Delicious Recipes to Help Lower Your Cholesterol* (New York: Clarkson Potter, 2004).

American Pain Society, *Guideline for the Management of Fibromyalgia Pain Syndrome in Adults and Children*, APS Clinical Practice Guidelines Series, No. 4 (Glenview, IL: American Pain Society, 2005).

Americans with Disabilities Act Handbook (Washington, DC: U.S. Equal Employment Opportunity Commission, 1992). [Employment resources; additional information at *www.disabilityinfo.gov*.

Aaron Antonovsky, *Unraveling the Mystery of Health: How People Manage Stress and Stay Well* (San Francisco: Jossey-Bass, 1987). Out of print.

Paul Arnstein, Margaret Caudill, Carol Lynn Mandle, A. Norris, and Ralph Beasley, "Self-Efficacy as a Mediator of the Relationship Between Pain Intensity, Disability and Depression in Chronic Pain Patients," *Pain, 81*: 483–491, 1999.

Robert Badgett, "Review: Injection Treatment Is Not Better than Placebo for Relieving Pain in Benign Chronic Low Back Pain," *Evidence-Based Medicine Online, 5*: 121, 2000. (Accessed 4/27/08)

Arthur J. Barsky and Emily C. Deans, *Feeling Better: A 6-Week Mind–Body Program to Ease Your Chronic Symptoms* (New York: HarperCollins, 2006).

Niels Becker, Per Sjogren, Per Bech, Alf Kornelius Olsen, and Jorgen Eriksen, "Treatment Outcome of Chronic Non-malignant Pain Patients Managed in a Danish Multidisciplinary Pain Centre Compared to General Practice: A Randomised Controlled Trial," *Pain, 84*: 203–211, 2000.

Lorna Bell and Eudora Seyfer, *Gentle Yoga* (Berkeley, CA: Celestial Arts, 1987).

Herbert Benson, *The Relaxation Response* (New York: HarperCollins, 2000).

Herbert Benson and Eileen Stuart, *The Wellness Book: The Comprehensive Guide to Maintaining Health and Treating Stress-Related Illness* (New York: Fireside, 1993).

Charles B. Berde, "Pain, Anxiety, Distress, and Suffering: Interrelated, But Not Interchangeable," *Journal of Pediatrics, 142*: 361–363, 2003.

Nicola Biller, Paul Arnstein, Margaret Caudill, Carol Wells-Federman, and Carolyn Guberman, "Predicting Completion of a Cognitive-Behavioral Pain Management Program by Initial Measures of a Chronic Pain Patient's Readiness for Change," *Clinical Journal of Pain, 16*(4): 352–359, 2000.

Joan Borysenko, *Minding the Body, Mending the Mind* (New York: Da Capo Press, 2007).

Carol Burckhardt, Don Goldenberg, Leslie Crofford, Robert Gerwin, Sue Gowans, Kenneth Jackson, et al., *Guideline for the Management of Fibromyalgia Syndrome Pain in Adults and Children*, APS Clinical Practice Guidelines Series, No. 4 (Glenview, IL: American Pain Society, 2005). Copies may be purchased from *www.ampainsoc.org*.

David Burns, *The Feeling Good Handbook* (New York: Plume, 1999).

David Burns, *Ten Days to Self-Esteem* (New York: Quill/William Morrow, 1999).

Margaret Caudill, Richard Schnable, Patricia Zuttermeister, Herbert Benson, and Richard Friedman, "Decreased Clinic Use by Chronic Pain Patients: Response to Behavioral Medicine Interventions," *Clinical Journal of Pain, 7*: 305–310, 1991.

Margaret A. Caudill-Slosberg, Lisa M. Schwartz, and Steven Woloshin, "Office Visits and Analgesic Prescriptions for Musculoskeletal Pain in US: 1980 vs. 2000," *Pain, 109*: 514–519, 2004.

John Chen and Tina T. Chen, *Chinese Medical Herbology and Pharmacology* (City of Industry, CA: Art of Medicine Press, 2004).

Robert Cialdini, *Influence: The Psychology of Persuasion* (New York: Collins, 2006).

Daniel O. Clegg, Domenic J. Reda, Crystal L. Harris, Marguerite A. Klein, James R. O'Dell, Michelle M. Hooper, et al., "Glucosamine, Chondroitin Sulfate, and the Two in Combination for Painful Knee Osteoarthritis," *New England Journal of Medicine, 354*: 795–808, 2006.

L. Gail Darlington, "Dietary Therapy for Arthritis," *Rheumatic Disease Clinics of North America, 17*: 273–285, 1991.

Gail Darlington and Linda Gamlin, *Diet and Arthritis* (North Pomfret, VT: Trafalgar Square, 1998).

Martha Davis, Matthew McKay, and Elizabeth Robbins Eshelman, *The Relaxation and Stress Reduction Workbook* (Oakland, CA: New Harbinger, 2000).

Thomas Delbanco, "Enriching the Doctor–Patient Relationship by Inviting the Patient's Perspective," *Annals of Internal Medicine, 116*: 414–418, 1992.

Ara DerMarderosian, Lawrence Liberti, John Beutler, and Constance Grauds (Eds.), *The Review of Natural Products, Fourth Edition* (New York: Lippincott Williams & Wilkins, 2005).

John Dimitrakov, Kurt Kroenke, William D. Steers, Charles Berde, David Zurakowski, Michael R. Freeman, et al., "Pharmacologic Management of Painful Bladder Syndrome/Interstitial Cystitis," *Archives of Internal Medicine, 167*(18): 1922–1929, 2007.

Johanna Dwyer, "Nutritional Remedies: Reasonable and Questionable," *Annals of Behavioral Medicine, 14*: 120–125, 1992.

L. D. Egbert, G. E. Battit, C. E. Welch, and M. K. Bartlett, "Reduction in Post-operative Pain by Encouragement and Instruction of Patients: A Study of Doctor–Patient Rapport," *New England Journal of Medicine, 270*: 825–827, 1964.

Paul Ekman, Robert Levenson, and Wallace Friesen, "Autonomic Nervous System Activity Distinguishes among Emotions," *Science, 221*: 1208–1210, 1983.

Albert Ellis, *How to Make Yourself Happy and Remarkably Less Disturbable* (Manassas Park, VA: Impact, 1999).

Patrick Fanning, *Visualization for Change* (Oakland, CA: New Harbinger Publications, 1994).

Fawzy I. Fawzy, Nancy Fawzy, Christine Hyun, Robert Elashoff, Donald Guthrie, John Fahey, et al., "Malignant Melanoma: Effects of an Early Structured Psychiatric Intervention, Coping, and Affective State on Recurrence and Survival 6 Years Later," *Archives of General Psychiatry, 50*: 681–688, 1993.

Howard L. Fields, *Pain Mechanisms and Management, Second Edition* (New York: McGraw-Hill, 2001).

Roger Fisher and William Ury, *Getting to Yes: Negotiating Agreement without Giving In* (New York: Penguin, 1991).

Beverly Flanigan, *Forgiving the Unforgivable: Overcoming the Bitter Legacy of Intimate Wounds* (New York: Wiley, 1992).

John Frank, Sandra Sinclair, Shielah Hogg-Johnson, Harry Shannon, Claire Bombadier, Dorcas Beaton, et al., "Preventing Disability from Work-Related Low-Back Pain," *Canadian Medical Journal, 158*: 1625–1631, 1998.

Shakti Gawain, *Creative Visualization* (New York: New World Library, 2002).

W. Doyle Gentry, *Anger Management for Dummies* (Hoboken, NJ: Wiley, 2007).

John Gormley and Juliette Hussey (Eds.), *Exercise Therapy: Prevention and Treatment of Disease* (Malden, MA: Blackwell, 2005).

Joerg Gruenwald, Thomas Brendler, and Christof Jaenicke (Eds.), *PDR for Herbal Medicines, Fourth Edition* (Montvale, NJ: Thomson Healthcare Inc., 2007).

Edward T. Hall, *Beyond Culture* (New York: Anchor, 1977).

Thich Nhat Hanh, *Anger: Wisdom for Cooling the Flames* (NewYork: Riverhead Books, 2001).

Thich Nhat Hanh, *The Miracle of Mindfulness: A Manual of Meditation* (Boston: Beacon Press, 1996).

Christopher W. Hoenig, *The Problem Solving Journey: Your Guide to Making Decisions and Getting Results* (Reading, MA: Basic Books, 2000).

Judith Horstman, *The Arthritis Foundation's Guide to Alternative Therapies* (Atlanta, GA: Arthritis Foundation, 1999).

Edmund Jacobson, *Progressive Relaxation* (Chicago: University of Chicago Press, 1938). Out of print.

Gary W. Jay, *Chronic Pain* (Boca Raton, FL: CRC Press, 2007).

Jon Kabat-Zinn, *Arriving at Your Own Door: 108 Lessons in Mindfulness* (New York: Hyperion, 2007).

Jon Kabat-Zinn, *Full Catastrophe Living: Using the Wisdom of Your Body and Mind to Face Stress, Pain, and Illness* (New York: Delacorte Press, 1990).

Adam Kahane and Peter M. Senge, *Solving Tough Problems: An Open Way of Talking, Listening, and Creating New Realities* (San Francisco: Berrett-Koehler, 2007).

Keith K. Karren, Brent Q. Hafen, Kathryn J. Frandsen, and Lee Smith, *Mind/Body Health: Effects of Attitudes, Emotions and Relationships, Third Edition* (Boston: Benjamin Cummings, 2006).

Jeff Keller, *Attitude Is Everything* (Tampa, FL: International Network Training Institute, 2007).

Jens Kjeldsen-Kragh et al., "Controlled Trial of Fasting and One-Year Vegetarian Diet in Rheumatoid Arthritis," *Lancet, 338*: 899–902, 1991.

Allen Klein, *The Healing Power of Humor* (Los Angeles: Tarcher, 1989).

Suzanne Kobasa, "Stressful Life Events, Personality and Health: An Inquiry into Hardiness," *Journal of Personality and Social Psychology, 37*: 1–11, 1979.

J. M. Kremer et al., "Effects of High Dose Fish Oil on Rheumatoid Arthritis after Stopping Nonsteroidal Anti-inflammatory Drugs: Clinical and Immune Correlates," *Arthritis and Rheumatology, 38*: 1107–1114, 1995.

Carol Krucoff, Mitchell Krucoff, and Adam Brill, *Healing Moves: How to Cure, Relieve, and Prevent Common Ailments with Exercise* (New York: Crown Publishers, 2000).

Loretta Laroche, *Life Is Not a Stress Rehearsal: Bringing Yesterday's Sane Wisdom into Today's Insane World* (New York: Broadway Books, 2001).

Richard S. Lazarus and Susan Folkman, *Stress, Appraisal, and Coping* (New York: Springer, 1984).

Kate Lorig and James Fries, *The Arthritis Helpbook: A Tested Self-Management Program for Coping with Arthritis and Fibromyalgia, Sixth Edition* (New York: Da Capo Press, 2006).

Mayo Clinic, *Mayo Clinic on Chronic Pain* (New York: Kensington, 1999).

Matthew McKay and Peter Rogers, *The Anger Control Workbook* (Oakland, CA: New Harbinger Publications, 2000).

M. A. Minor and M. K. Sanford, "Physical Interventions in the Management of Pain in Arthritis," *Arthritis Care and Research, 6*: 197–206, 1993.

James Moore, Kate Lorig, Michael VanKorff, Virginia Gonzalez, and Diane Laurent, *The Back Pain Helpbook* (Reading, MA: Perseus Books, 1999).

David Morris, *The Culture of Pain* (Berkeley: University of California Press, 1991).

Miriam Nelson, Kristin Baker, and Ronenn Roubenoff, with Lawrence Lindner, *Strong Women and Men Beat Arthritis* (New York: G. P. Putnam's Sons, 2002).

Miriam Nelson, Wendy Wray, and Sarah Wernick, *Strong Women Stay Young* (New York: Bantam, 2005).

Portia Nelson, *There's a Hole in My Sidewalk* (Hillsboro, OR: Beyond Words, 1994).

Samara Joy Nielsen and Barry M. Popkin. "Patterns and Trends in Food Portion Sizes, 1977–1998," *Journal of the American Medical Association, 289*(4): 450–453, 2003.

D. C. Nordstrom et al., "Alpha Linoleic Acid in the Treatment of Rheumatoid Arthritis: A Double Blind, Placebo Controlled and Randomized Study: Flaxseed vs. Safflower Oil," *Rheumatology International, 14*: 231–234, 1995.

Nutrition Action Healthletter. For subscription information, write to the Center for Science in the Public Interest, P.O. Box 96611, Washington DC 20090-6611; e-mail: *circ@cspinet.org*, or order online at *www.cspinet.org*.

Judith K. Ockene, "Physician-Delivered Interventions for Smoking Cessation," *Preventive Medicine, 16*: 723–737, 1987.

Robert Ornstein, *Evolution of Consciousness* (New York: Touchstone, 1992).

Robert Ornstein, *The Psychology of Consciousness, 2nd Ed.* (New York: Penguin, 1996).

Robert Ornstein and David Sobel, *The Healing Brain* (Los Altos, CA: Malor Books, 1999).

Robert Ornstein and David Sobel, *Healthy Pleasures* (New York: Da Capo Press, 1990).

Richard Panush, "Does Food Cause or Cure Arthritis?" *Rheumatic Disease Clinics of North America, 17*: 259–272, 1991.

A. M. Pearson, E. A. Blood, J. W. Frymoyer, H. Herkowitz, W. A. Abdu, R. Woodward, et al., "SPORT Lumbar Intervertebral Disk Herniation and Back Pain: Does Treatment, Location, or Morphology Matter?" *Spine, 33*(4): 428–435, 2008.

James Pennebaker, *Opening Up: The Healing Power of Expressing Emotions* (New York: Guilford Press, 1997).

Jean A. T. Pennington and Helen Nichols Church, *Bowes and Church's Food Values of Portions Commonly Used, Thirteenth Edition* (New York: Harper & Row, 1980).

Portion Size. Research to Practice Series, No. 2: Portion Size (Atlanta: Centers for Disease Control and Prevention, 2006). Available at *www.cdc.gov/nccdphp/dnpa/nutrition/pdf/portion_size_research.pdf.*

Reynolds Price, *A Whole New Life* (New York: Scribner, 2000).

Cynthia Radnitz, "Food Triggered Migraine: A Critical Review," *Annals of Behavioral Medicine, 12*: 51–64, 1990.

James Rainville, David Ahern, Linda Phalen, Lisa Childs, and Robin Sutherland, "The Association of Pain with Physical Activities in Chronic Low Back Pain," *Spine, 17*: 1060–1064, 1992.

R. C. Rinaldi, E. M. Steindler, B. B. Wilford, and D. Goodwin, "Clarification and Standardization of Substance Terminology," *Journal of the American Medical Association, 259*: 555–557, 1988.

Carol Ann Rinzler, *Nutrition for Dummies, Fourth Edition* (Hoboken, NJ: Wiley, 2006).

James M. Rippe and Ann Ward, *Rockport's Complete Book of Fitness Walking* (New York: Prentice-Hall Press, 1989).

Carl Rogers, *Client-Centered Therapy: Its Current Practice, Implications, and Theory* (Boston: Houghton Mifflin, 1951). Out of print.

Daniel Rooks, Shiva Gautam, Matthew Romeling, Martha Cross, Diana Stratigakis, Brittany Evans, et al., "Group Exercise, Education, and Combination Self-Management in Women with Fibromyalgia: A Randomized Trial," *Archives of Internal Medicine, 167*: 2192–2200, 2007.

Marshall Rosenberg and Arun Gandhi, *Nonviolent Communication: A Language of Life* (Encinitas, CA: PuddleDancer Press, 2005).

Larry A. Samovar, Richard E. Porter, and Edwin R. McDaniel, *Communication between Cultures* (Wadsworth Series in Communication Studies) (Boston, MA: Thomson Learning, 2006).

Anne Wilson Schaef, *Meditations for Women Who Do Too Much, Revised Edition* (San Francisco: HarperOne, 2004).

Niall Scott and Jonathan Seglow, *Altruism* (New York: Open University Press, 2007).

Martin Seligman, *Learned Optimism: How to Change Your Mind and Your Life* (New York: Vintage, 2006).

Idries Shah, *The Pleasantries of the Incredible Mulla Nasrudin* (London: Octagon Press, 1983).

Idries Shah, *Reflections* (London: Octagon Press, 1983).

Idries Shah, *The Subtleties of the Inimitable Mulla Nasrudin* and *The Exploits of the Incomparable Mulla Nasrudin* (London: Octagon Press, 1989).

David Sobel and Robert Ornstein, *The Healthy Mind Healthy Body Handbook* (Los Altos, CA: Malor Books, 1997).

Jenny Steinmetz, Jon Blankenship, Linda Brown, Deborah Hall, and Grace Miller, *Managing Stress Before It Manages You* (Palo Alto, CA: Bull, 1980).

Deborah Tannen, *The Power of Talk: Who Gets Heard and Why (HBR OnPoint Enhanced Edition)*, e-document download available through Amazon.com, January 5, 2008.

Deborah Tannen, *That's Not What I Meant! How Conversational Style Makes or Breaks Relationships* (New York: Ballantine Books, 1992).

Deborah Tannen, *You Just Don't Understand: Women and Men in Conversation* (New York: Harper Paperbacks, 2001).

Madisyn Taylor, *Daily OM: Inspirational Thoughts for a Happy, Healthy and Fulfilling Day* (Carlsbad, CA: Hay House, 2008).

Beverly Thorn, *Cognitive Therapy for Chronic Pain: A Step-by-Step Guide* (New York: Guilford Press, 2004).

Tufts University Health & Nutrition Letter. Information online at *tuftshealthletter.com* or write to P.O. Box 420235, Palm Coast, FL 32142.

Dennis Turk, Donald Meichenbaum, and Myles Genest, *Pain and Behavioral Medicine: A Cognitive-Behavioral Perspective* (New York: Guilford Press, 1985).

Dennis C. Turk and Frits Winter, *The Pain Survival Guide: How to Reclaim Your Life* (Washington, DC: American Psychological Association, 2005).

U.S. Department of Health and Human Services, Centers for Disease Control and Prevention, National Center for Chronic Disease Prevention and President's Council on Physical Fitness, *Physical Activity and Health: A Report of the Surgeon General* (Sudbury, MA: Jones and Bartlett, 1998).

Patrick Wall and Steven Rose (Eds.), *Pain: The Science of Suffering* (New York: Columbia University Press, 2000).

Carol Warfield and Zahid Bajwa, *Principles and Practice of Pain Medicine, Second Edition* (New York: McGraw-Hill, 2004).

Hope S. Warshaw and George Blackburn, *The Restaurant Companion: A Guide to Healthier Eating Out* (Chicago: Surrey Books, 1995).

Andrew Weil, *Eating Well for Optimum Health: The Essential Guide to Food, Diet, and Nutrition* (New York: Knopf, 2000).

Andrew Weil, *Health and Healing: Understanding Conventional and Alternative Medicine* (Boston: Houghton Mifflin, 1998).

J. N. Weinstein, T. D. Tosteson, J. D. Lurie, A. N. Tosteson, E. Blood, B. Hanscom, et al., "Surgical versus Nonsurgical Therapy for Lumbar Spinal Stenosis," *New England Journal of Medicine, 358*(8): 794–810, 2008.

Hendria Weisinger, *Dr. Weisinger's Anger Workout Book* (New York: Quill, 1985).

Walter C. Willett and P. J. Skerrett, *Eat, Drink, and Be Healthy: The Harvard Medical School Guide to Healthy Eating* (New York: Free Press, 2005).

Redford B. Williams and Virginia Williams, *Anger Kills: Seventeen Strategies for Controlling the Hostility That Can Harm Your Health* (New York: Harper Paperbacks, 1998).

Denise Winn, *The Manipulated Mind: Brainwashing, Conditioning and Manipulation* (Los Altos, CA: Malor Books, 2000).

Frederick Wolfe et al., "The American College of Rheumatology 1990 Criteria for the Classification of Fibromyalgia," *Arthritis and Rheumatism, 33*: 160–172, 1990.

Index

About the Author

Margaret A. Caudill, MD, PhD, MPH, is a board-certified internist and a Diplomate of Pain Medicine. For more than 25 years, Dr. Caudill has worked to improve the lives of people with chronic illness through medical treatments that address both mind and body. She has researched, written, and lectured extensively on mind–body medicine and the biopsychosocial treatment of pain. Currently, she is Instructor of Anesthesiology at Dartmouth Hitchcock Medical Center's Pain Management Center, Lebanon, New Hampshire, and Adjunct Associate Professor of Clinical and Family Medicine at Dartmouth Medical School.

Perforated Worksheets
and Other Materials

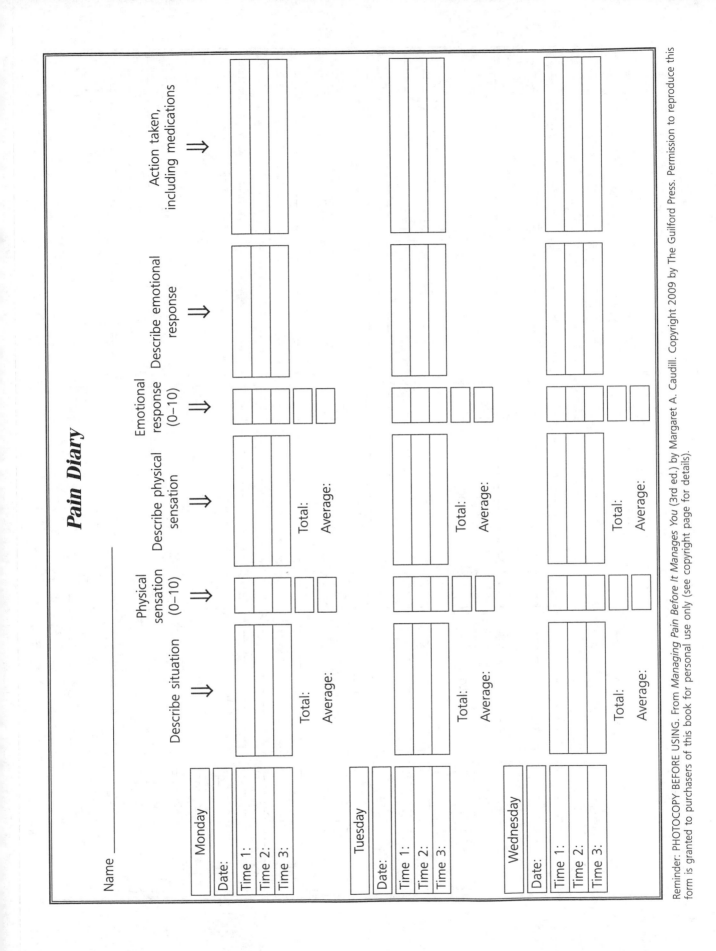

Pain Diary

Pain Diary (cont.)

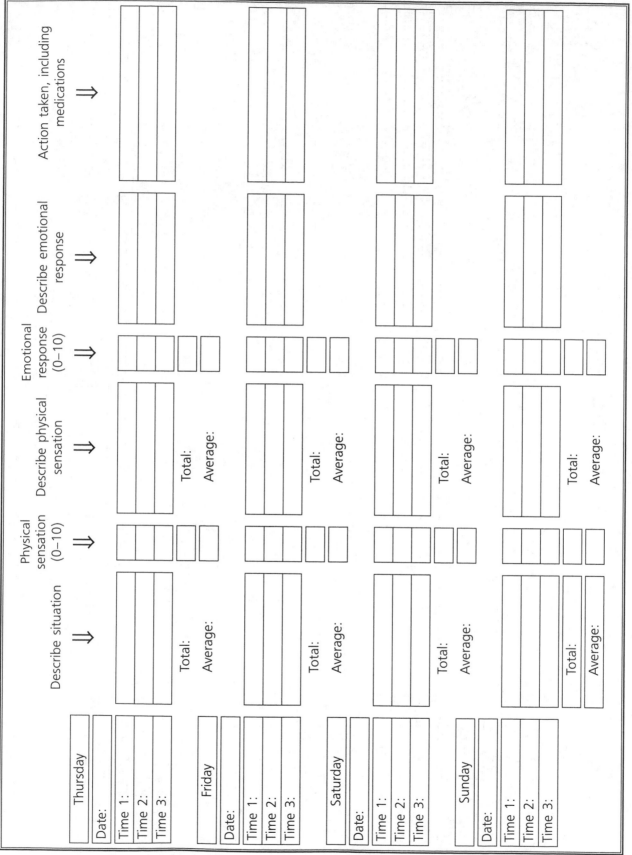

Describe situation ⟹
Physical sensation (0–10) ⟹
Describe physical sensation ⟹
Emotional response (0–10) ⟹
Describe emotional response ⟹
Action taken, including medications ⟹

Thursday
Date:
Time 1:
Time 2:
Time 3:
Total:
Average:

Friday
Date:
Time 1:
Time 2:
Time 3:
Total:
Average:

Saturday
Date:
Time 1:
Time 2:
Time 3:
Total:
Average:

Sunday
Date:
Time 1:
Time 2:
Time 3:
Total:
Average:

Medication List

Name _____

List last updated _____

Medication	How is it prescribed?	Pill dose?	Total dose per day	What's it for?	Morning	Midday	Evening	Bedtime	Prescribed by	Over the counter? (Check if yes)

See sample Medication List, p. 44.

Relaxation Response Technique Diary

Complete the following weekly RR Diary. Next to each category indicate the appropriate information about your daily practice. Use this diary for the first 3 weeks to reinforce practice.

Date							
Time started							
Time stopped							
Place							
Position (lying down, sitting)							
Degree of relaxation at end (0–10) 0 = very relaxed 10 = very tense							
Effects on pain? Decrease = D Increase = I No change = NC							
Method (tape, exercise, visualization, other)							

Were there any problems that prevented you from practicing the RR daily? How can you solve the problem(s)? _____

_____

_____

_____

_____

_____

_____

_____

Increasing Activities Worksheet

Date: _____ Name: _____

Make a list of activities that increase your pain and those that decrease your pain (refer to Chapter 4).

Activities that increase my pain	**Activities that decrease my pain**
Example: Washing dishes (standing)	Paying bills (sitting)

_____   _____

_____   _____

_____   _____

_____   _____

_____   _____

Can you *delegate* any of the activities associated with pain increases? (For example, bringing dirty laundry to the washing machine.) Star (*) the ones you can.

Delegate one activity this week. It will be _____

Choose one "increase pain" activity from your list and time how long it takes to increase pain level by 2 points. Then choose a "decrease pain" activity and time how long it takes for the pain to decrease again. Alternate between activities that increase and decrease your pain.

Example: Pain ↑ Activity = Wash dishes   Pain ↓ Activity = Pay bills

Wash dishes (10 mins.)   Sort bills from mail (15 mins.)

Wash dishes (10 mins.)   Write checks (15 mins.)

Wash dishes (10 mins.)   Address envelopes (10 mins.)

Activity that increases pain	**Activity that decreases pain**

_____   _____

_____   _____

_____   _____

_____   _____

Can you *adapt* any of the above activities so that they can be performed more easily? What would be some of the adaptations? (For example: sitting to fold laundry or peel vegetables; lying down to call a friend or listen to a book on tape; opening cabinet door under kitchen sink so that you can rest one foot on the shelf; putting bowls in sink to stir ingredients)

_____

_____

_____

_____

Daily Record of Automatic Thoughts (Self-Talk)

Date	Situation	Automatic thoughts	Physical response	Emotional response	Cognitive distortion	Changed thought

Food Diary Instructions

Time started: The time of day that you begin eating a meal.

Food/beverage: Record everything you eat and drink. Note such things as whether the food or beverage contained a sweetener substitute or whether it was a new product for you. Are you eating five servings of fruits and vegetables and six servings of grain products (including whole grains) per day?

Quantity: The amount that you ate or drank (e.g., 1 cup, 8 oz. glass) or the plate portion (½, ¼ of the dinner plate).

Time ended: The time at which you ended the meal you were recording. (If a number of your meals last 10 minutes or less, maybe you should consider eating more slowly.)

You may have to keep a food diary for many weeks before you see a relationship between foods and pain patterns.

Food Diary

Date: _____ Name: _____

Time started	Food/beverage	Quantity	Time ended

Weekly Feedback Sheet

Name: _____

Date: _____ Reporting for week of: _____

1. Record the daily averages of your physical sensation and emotional response below:

	Day 1	Day 2	Day 3	Day 4	Day 5	Day 6	Day 7	Weekly average
Physical sensation:	____	____	____	____	____	____	____	____
Emotional response:	____	____	____	____	____	____	____	____

   If this is your first session, record your pain level now (on a scale of 0–10): ____

2. Over the past week, has your *physical sensation*:

   Improved ____   Stayed the same ____   Become worse ____

   Why do you think that your *physical sensation* has improved, stayed the same, or become worse?

   _____

   _____

   Over the past week, has your *emotional response*:

   Improved ____   Stayed the same ____   Become worse ____

   Why do you think that your *emotional response* has improved, stayed the same, or become worse?

   _____

   _____

3. List all medication you are taking:

Name of medication	Dosage (mg)	Frequency*
_____	_____	_____
_____	_____	_____
_____	_____	_____
_____	_____	_____
_____	_____	_____
_____	_____	_____
_____	_____	_____

   *How many times per day or per week do you take each medication?

   If you take opioids, how many pills did you take for this week? ____

4. Did you receive any other pain treatments this week—for example, nerve blocks, physical therapy, acupuncture, etc.? _____

_____

_____

5. How many times this week did you do the following?

Relaxation response techniques _____   Mini-relaxations _____

6. For how long and how often did you do physical exercise this week?

Aerobic _____   Time _____   How often? _____

Stretching _____   Time _____   How often? _____

Strengthening _____   Time _____   How often? _____

7. What goal did you set for the week? _____
Did you accomplish it? (Y/N) _____   If you did not accomplish it, can you come up with a contingency plan that might help you succeed by identifying the obstacle and a solution to the obstacle?

Obstacle	Solution
_____	_____
_____	_____
_____	_____
_____	_____

8. Where did you find your pleasure this week? _____
_____
_____
_____

9. Do you have any questions or problems? _____
_____
_____
_____

10. To health care professionals: Is there any other information you wish to collect? Fill in before copying.
_____
_____
_____
_____
_____
_____
_____
_____

Please Do Not Disturb

I'm relaxing per my doctor's orders

Letter to Health Care Professionals

Dear Health Care Professional:

Managing Pain Before It Manages You is a practical, patient-oriented workbook. It provides information on basic pain mechanisms, medical treatment of chronic pain, and multiple cognitive behavioral skills that can assist coping and functioning. This book can be used by patients alone, but it can be even more effective if supported by a health care professional who can guide the patient through the program and reinforce the book's information. The workbook was originally written to supplement a 10-visit group medical program for chronic pain management, but it can be used in individual therapy as well.

If you are a physician, nurse practitioner, or physician assistant, this book can supplement the pharmacological, interventional, and surgical treatments recommended to patients with chronic pain.

If you are a psychologist, social worker, or nurse, this workbook offers a complete, self-guided cognitive behavioral therapy program for your clients or patients. It may be used in patient education, in conjunction with other medical therapies, and in psychotherapy. Patients can use the workbook independently or as a formal 8- to 10-week individual or group program.

Efficacy of This Approach

A growing body of evidence supports the biopsychosocial treatment of chronic pain. The biopsychosocial approach is further supported by evidence-based treatment guidelines such as those that can be found in the *Cochrane Database of Systematic Reviews* (*www3.interscience.wiley.com/cgi-in/mrwhome/106568753/HOME*), *BMJ Clinical Evidence* (*www.clinicalevidence.com/ceweb*), the U.S. government's Effective Health Care Program *effectivehealthcare.ahrq.gov*), and through such evidence-based search engines as the TRIP Database (*www.tripdatabase.com*).

The best approach to chronic pain syndromes is a comprehensive one that includes a thorough history and physical exam to understand the source of pathology or pain etiology, a stepwise approach to address the multiple sources of pain and distress, and repeated reassessment to assure responsiveness to treatment. Chronic pain is either perpetuated through central nervous system mechanisms (nonnociceptive) or related to underlying chronic painful diseases (nociceptive). Both types of pain are essentially incurable at this time unless the underlying pathology can be eliminated. As such, both are benefited by biological, psychological, and sociological therapies that reduce symptoms, increase activity, and assist patients in coping with chronic illness and managing their symptoms. The materials presented in this book are grounded in the principles of chronic disease management. They are a synthesis of medical and behavioral approaches to symptom and disease management that have been shown to decrease symptoms and decrease clinic utilization (Caudill et al., 1991; Becker et al., 2000). Furthermore, this intervention program can increase self-efficacy, an important mediator of pain-related disability and depression symptoms (Arnstein et al., 1999).

The Professional's Role in Facilitating this Program

> Those who do not feel pain, seldom think that it is felt.
> —*Samuel Johnson, MD, 1708–1784*

Progress has been made in the understanding of pain mechanisms but there is much that remains a mystery. While there is no objective measure of pain at this time, it is important to believe patients who report their pain experience. It is important for you and your patient to acknowledge that although living in pain is a challenge, there are many things that can be done to decrease symptoms and improve quality of life. If you do not feel comfortable evaluating and treating chronic pain, it is your obligation to refer the patient to someone who can.

Many health care professionals feel unsure about how to evaluate or treat pain. Such uncertainty has helped to drive the inappropriate prescribing of opioids in the past decade (Caudill-Slosberg et al., 2004). At the same time, there has been a dramatic increase in pharmaceutical advertising in popular media as well as to physicians. This has created unrealistic demands for pharmacologic cures by patients who understandably can feel quite desperate to be pain free. It is therefore crucial that the health professional and the patient understand the proposed pain mechanisms and treatment rationale described in Chapter 2 of this workbook. This information can help explain both the limits of pharmaceutical, surgical, and interventional therapies and the need for physical activity, good nutrition, and effective coping strategies.

Assessing and Encouraging Patient Readiness for Change

Teaching an appreciation of the biopsychosocial process at the time of the initial evaluation lends validity to treatments such as cognitive behavioral therapies. Explore what other symptoms patients are experiencing in addition to their pain. The professional can help identify stress-related symptoms such as fatigue, memory problems, irritable bowel, muscle tension, shortness of breath, palpitations, irritability, and insomnia. Questions about the patient's psychosocial history can help identify other influencing issues and provide more mind–body connections for discussion. For example:

- "What activities have you changed because of your pain?" Humans are incredibly adaptable and are quite capable of using denial for coping. Detailing what work and leisure activities have been curtailed inside and outside the home offers evidence for the magnitude of pain complaints.
- "Where do you get your emotional support? Who or what helps you to problem-solve?" Behavioral medicine research has documented the positive power of support through close friends, spouses, and religious affiliation. However, many patients with chronic pain suffer isolation and despair.
- "In addition to your pain and the problems it causes, what other stresses do you have to cope with right now?" This can be a very revealing question. The losses incurred from unemployment or decreased work capacity alone can have economic, social, and self-esteem consequences of enormous importance.
- "Have you ever been physically, emotionally, or sexually abused? Have you experienced a trauma?" There is a very high positive response to this question in my practice. Such histories are important to uncover since they influence how to teach relaxation skills. Patients with a history of trauma or abuse may require individual treatment to distinguish the emotional consequences of these events from similar experiences common in chronic pain patients, such as feeling vulnerable or out of control, or that one is not believed by others.

- "Do you have any fears or concerns about your pain? What do you think is going on?" The majority of patients have ideas (or fears) about the source or cause of their pain. For obvious reasons, addressing these concerns may go a long way in getting them to recognize their part in pain management.
- "What do you want to get from your visit today?" This sends the message that the patient has a right to have expectations for a visit. It is also a good starting point in clarifying unrealistic expectations. It can be the perfect opening to discuss the roles of the health care professional and patient in reaching a common goal.
- "If I can't cure you today, what would be the next best thing?" This question stems from a common response of many patients to the last question. They will say, "You don't understand, doctor, I don't want my pain, so why would I want to manage it?" This again allows for discussion of the nature and reality of chronic, persistent pain. Early in treatment many people feel that acceptance of pain management is a condemnation to a life of pain even if a cure comes along. They somehow think they will be excluded because they have accepted their pain. This misunderstanding is important to clarify. Acceptance is dealing with the here and now; pain may be mandatory, but the suffering is definitely optional.

These questions can quickly give you an overview of an individual's pain experience and lay the groundwork for establishing that pain is both stressful and affected by stress. It also sends the message that you are concerned about the pain and the person in pain. Listening to the patient's responses to these questions helps set up realistic treatment expectations and orients treatment to the patient's level of understanding.

Patients in precontemplation (Biller et al., 2000) who have not thought about the relationship between behavior and pain can be asked just to read Chapters 1 through 5 of the workbook, without doing the exercises described. They can also begin keeping a pain diary, as described in Chapter 1, which will help them focus on just how their pain is affected by their daily activities and mood.

Patients are most ready to start *using* this workbook when they can acknowledge (1) that changing their behavior may help them cope with or manage their pain or (2) that they need new skills to handle the physical, emotional, and cognitive effects of pain on their lives.

Guiding Patients through the Workbook

When patients are ready, this workbook can provide a guide for change. It is helpful to set a start date with the patient to begin implementing this program. It is also useful to review patient's goals. This demonstrates your interest and insures that the patient's goals are realistic and achievable.

Patients consistently report the benefits of the relaxation response technique, pacing activities, exercise, challenging negative self-talk, and diary keeping. If time is limited, focusing on these skills may be most productive. Otherwise, a chapter a week is a realistic pace to set.

With each week and each chapter, more observations and skills are added to the coping repertoire. Encourage patients to keep using and adding to the skills—with the hope of achieving a synergism—not just to do them one at a time.

To encourage action, ask at follow-up visits what patients are learning from their diary keeping, relaxation response techniques, and activity pacing. Because the cognitive therapy skills can begin to challenge some basic assumptions and beliefs, patients may be reluctant to do the writing exercises. These are crucial to changing cognitive distortions and ineffective patterns of thinking. Encourage patients to bring these exercise sheets to their follow-up appointments or to keep a journal. Journaling can help patients become more comfortable with what goes on inside the mind and how it reacts to the world. Growing self-awareness can gently move patients into action. This movement toward maintenance of action over time is essential for behavioral change to occur and set the stage for a new standard of living.

The sequence of chapters in this workbook reflects the way the program is taught. The arrangement of topics is geared toward encouraging patient adherence to the program through the gradual build-up of pain management skills. Techniques that are easier to learn and provide more immediate results—such as relaxation response techniques and exercise—are presented first. Once patients have successfully adopted these skills, they receive positive inducement to continue with the more complex techniques—ones requiring long-term practice, introspection, and self-reflection—taught in later chapters.

Pain Flare-Up Management and Maintenance

Chapter 10 of the workbook addresses relapse prevention and pain flare-up management. Whichever technique the patient chooses to employ, either "coping with stages of pain" or the "panic plan," a copy of the plan should be kept in his or her record and periodically updated. Referral to the plan can then be made should he or she experience a pain flare-up. However, if the patient insists that a particular pain flare-up is different from what he or she usually experiences, a reassessment is necessary to rule out other developments. I have found that once patients become active participants in pain management through this program, they are the best judges of their own pain experience.

From here on, periodic inquiries about maintenance of skills such as relaxation response techniques (Chapter 3), mini-relaxations (Chapter 3), pacing activities (Chapter 4), strategies for response to negative emotional states (Chapters 5 and 6), reduced caffeine consumption (Chapter 7), and communication skills (Chapter 8) will also serve to reinforce behavioral change maintenance. If patients have stopped practicing these skills and are having increased difficulty with pain management, it may be necessary for you to identify the specific problems holding them back. For example, has a setback occurred because the patient was secretly hoping this program would cure his or her pain, and it didn't? Did the patient stop the program because it was going so well it didn't seem necessary anymore? Or is a separate life crisis distracting him or her from the pain management program? Once you have determined what issues are involved, you can set a date for the patient to get back into the program and then reinstitute a schedule of periodic checks on his or her skills practice.

A Final Note

I cannot emphasize enough what a rewarding experience it is to see people change, improve their quality of life, and feel more empowered in the face of some of the most difficult pain problems. It is critical to start from where the patients are in terms of their level of information, beliefs, and readiness to consider new directions in behavior and lifestyle practices. Your important role in facilitating this process will have its own rewards.

Margaret A. Caudill, MD, PhD, MPH
Dartmouth Medical School
Hanover, NH

References

Paul Arnstein, Margaret Caudill, Carol Lynn Mandle, A. Norris, and Ralph Beasley, "Self-Efficacy as a Mediator of the Relationship Between Pain Intensity, Disability and Depression in Chronic Pain Patients," *Pain*, *81*: 483–491, 1999.

Niels Becker, Per Sjogren, Per Bech, Alf Kornelius Olsen, and Jorgen Eriksen, "Treatment Outcome of Chronic Nonmalignant Pain Patients Managed in a Danish Multidisciplinary Pain Centre Compared to General Practice: A Randomised Controlled Trial," *Pain, 84*: 203–211, 2000.

Nicola Biller, Paul Arnstein, Margaret Caudill, Carol Wells-Federman, and Carolyn Guberman, "Predicting Completion of a Cognitive-Behavioral Pain Management Program by Initial Measures of a Chronic Pain Patient's Readiness for Change. *Clinical Journal of Pain*, *16*(4): 352–359, 2000.

Margaret Caudill, Richard Schnable, Patricia Zuttenneister, Herbert Benson, and Richard Friedman, "Decreased Clinic Use by Chronic Pain Patients: Response to Behavioral Medicine Intervention," *Clinical Journal of Pain, 7*: 305–310, 1991.

Margaret Caudill-Slosberg, Lisa Schwartz, and Steven Woloshin, "Office Visits and Analgesic Prescriptions for Musculoskeletal Pain in US: 1980 vs. 2000," *Pain, 109*: 514–519, 2004.

Dennis Turk, Donald Meichenbaum, and Myles Genest, *Pain and Behavioral Medicine: A Cognitive-Behavioral Perspective* (New York: Guilford Press, 1985).